Mastering the

USMLE

Step 2 CS
(Clinical Skills Examination)

Notice

Medicine is an ever-changing science. As new research and clinical experience broaden our knowledge, changes in treatment and drug therapy are required. The authors and the publisher of this work have checked with sources believed to be reliable in their efforts to provide information that is complete and generally in accord with the standards accepted at the time of publication. However, in view of the possibility of human error or changes in medical sciences, neither the authors nor the publisher nor any other party who has been involved in the preparation or publication of this work warrants that the information contained herein is in every respect accurate or complete, and they disclaim all responsibility for any errors or omissions or for the results obtained from use of the information contained in this work. Readers are encouraged to confirm the information contained herein with other sources. For example and in particular, readers are advised to check the product information sheet included in the package of each drug they plan to administer to be certain that the information contained in this work is accurate and that changes have not been made in the recommended dose or in the contraindications for administration. This recommendation is of particular importance in connection with new or infrequently used drugs.

Mastering the

USMLE

3rd edition

Step 2 CS
(Clinical Skills Examination)

Jo-Ann Reteguiz, M.D., F.A.C.P.

VICE-CHAIR FOR EDUCATION
DEPARTMENT OF MEDICINE
UNIVERSITY OF MEDICINE AND DENTISTRY
OF NEW JERSEY–NEW JERSEY MEDICAL SCHOOL
NEWARK, NEW JERSEY

ILLUSTRATIONS BY MOIRA MCDONOUGH

McGraw-Hill
Medical Publishing Division

New York / Chicago / San Francisco / Lisbon
London / Madrid / Mexico City / New Delhi
San Juan / Singapore / Sydney / Toronto

Mastering the USMLE Step 2 CS (Clinical Skills Examination), Third edition

6 7 8 9 10 QVS/QVS 1 9 8 7 6 5 4 3

ISBN 0-07-144334-7

This book was set in New Baskerville by Circle Graphics.
The editors were Catherine A. Johnson and Mary E. Bele.
The production supervisor was Richard Ruzycka.
The cover designer was Aimee Nordin.
The index was prepared by Andover Publishing Services.

This book is printed on acid-free paper.

Library of Congress Cataloging-in-Publication Data

Reteguiz, Jo-Ann.
    Mastering the USMLE Step 2 CS (Clinical Skills Examination) / Jo-Ann Reteguiz ;
illustrations by Moira McDonough. — 3rd ed.
      p. ; cm.
    Rev. ed. of: Mastering the OSCE, Objective Structured Clinical Examination and CSA,
Clinical Skills Assessment. 2001.
    Includes bibliographical references and index.
    ISBN 0-07-144334-7
    1. Diagnosis—Examinations, questions, etc. 2. Medical history taking—Examinations,
questions, etc. 3. Physical diagnosis—Examinations, questions, etc. 4. Clinical
competence—Examinations, questions, etc. 5. Physicians—Licenses—United
States—Examinations—Study guides. I. Title: USMLE Step 2 CS (Clinical Skills
Examination). II. Reteguiz, Jo-Ann. Mastering the OSCE, Objective Structured Clinical
Examination and CSA, Clinical Skills Assessment. III. Title.
   [DNLM: 1. Physical Examination—methods—Problems and Exercises. 2. Clinical
Competence—Problems and Exercises. 3. Diagnosis—Problems and Exercises. 4. Medical
History Taking—methods—Problems and Exercises. WB 18.2 R437m 2005]
RC71.R48 2005
616.07'5'076—dc22
                                            2004058197

To my mother, Iris, and father, George, whose love and encouragement give special meaning to every journey.

—J.R.

Contents

WHO WILL FIND THIS BOOK USEFUL:

■ The U.S. medical student required to pass a clerkship standardized patient examination when rotating through the disciplines of internal medicine, family medicine, ob/gyn, pediatrics, psychiatry, emergency medicine, and surgery.

■ The U.S. medical student required to pass a senior year multidisciplinary clinical skills examination prior to graduation.

■ International and U.S. medical graduates who must pass the Step 2 CS for licensure or ECFMG certification. This book will guide physicians through the standardized patient examination.

■ The graduate who has failed the Step 2 CS and must retake the examination.

HOW THIS BOOK WILL HELP YOU:

■ Mastering the USMLE Step 2 CS Examination focuses your interviewing and physical examination skills so you are able to finish test stations in the required time limit.

■ It explains how you can develop the hidden "checklist" each standardized patient is using at every test station.

■ It sharpens your interpersonal skills to improve overall clinical performance.

■ It reveals the pitfalls of the standardized patient examination and shows how to avoid them.

■ It allows you to practice your approach to the standardized patient examination at home using "real" standardized patient cases.

■ It gives you the confidence and experience you need to do your best in any standardized patient interaction.

■ It allows you to practice writing clear, organized, and accurate patient notes. Over fifty patient notes are provided to help you develop proficiency in synthesizing and analyzing data.

■ It offers great practice for physicians and students when they interact with "real life" patients in the future.

HOW TO USE THIS BOOK:

■ Read the information in the early chapters to learn how to prepare for the standardized patient examination.

■ Understand the role of the standardized patient. This layperson is often the only person evaluating your performance.

■ Learn how to develop, accurately and quickly, the checklist used by the standardized patient at each test station. The examination requires you to develop a specific strategy based on the "hidden" checklist. If you can develop the checklist mentally before the actual interaction, the test becomes easy.

■ Learn how to write a patient note with complete and relevant information. A good patient note demonstrates your ability to interpret data and manage patients appropriately.

■ Use the more than fifty standardized patient cases in this book to practice and grade your checklist developing skills and your patient note writing ability.

■ Review Pearls:

 Patient Note Pearl

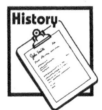 History-Taking Pearl

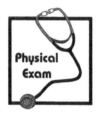 Physical Examination Pearl

Background

The "gold standard" by which physician competence is measured has eluded medical educators for over a century. Early in the history of medicine, senior physicians mentored and graded their students, but the limitations of this subjective process were obvious. Specialty boards began using the oral examination, which provided more accurate information about a physician's clinical problem-solving skills and fund of knowledge, but these were not reliable or standardized. Excellent or poor performance on the oral examination reflected the good luck of being asked to discuss a clinical problem seen during training or the bad luck of being asked about a case one had never seen.

In the middle of the twentieth century, using multiple choice questions (MCQ) on a written examination became the method for physician evaluation and, for over four decades, medical schools and licensure bureaus relied on "the written" to assess whether a physician or student was competent. Educators soon realized that, even though MCQ examinations were standardized and reliable, they lacked validity. It was clear that an 80 percent score on the written examination did not mean that the examinee knew 80 percent of all of medicine. Was the paper-and-pencil examination the best way of judging competence? Could educators say that "the written" accurately simulated the tasks future physicians would be expected to perform in "real life" medicine?

In 1963, at the University of Southern California, Dr. Howard Barrows trained a healthy artist's model to portray a paralyzed patient with multiple sclerosis. In this way, neurology students learned about the disease from a "real" patient instead of a textbook. This was the first standardized patient encounter.

In 1964, Barrows and Abrahamson suggested using standardized patients in a test format to assess student performance in medical school. Using "real" clinical situations and "real" patients, one could assess how students used their knowledge and skills when faced with realistic challenges, rather than trying to infer performance from a standardized written test. This was the beginning of the standardized patient examination.

Over the last forty years, the standardized patient examination has evolved into an important tool for the teaching and assessment of medical students and physicians. It has gained acceptance as a requirement for licensure and medical school graduation. In a world where astronauts practice simulated space exploration before "real" flight and computers simulate everything from golf to warfare, it was only a matter of time before medicine, too, required simulated practice and assessment before allowing a physician to encounter the "real" clinical situation.

Preface

The purpose of this Step 2 CS review book is to help medical students and physicians faced with the stress of taking a new-format examination become more comfortable with the standardized patient encounter.

As the Medicine Clerkship Course Director at the University of Medicine and Dentistry of New Jersey-New Jersey Medical School, I successfully integrated a standardized patient examination for over 1500 medical students. After 7 years of standardized patient test writing, training, implementation, and grading, I realized that a student could perform poorly due to nervousness and inexperience with this kind of examination. Students would often approach me for tips and advice on how to improve their performance on the standardized patient examination.

The unique qualities of the standardized patient examination make it, understandably, a stressful experience. In less than 15 minutes, a student must interview and examine a patient and accurately formulate a differential diagnosis and plan. At each test station, the examinee must demonstrate excellent communication skills and remarkable composure. In 10 minutes, the student must write a complete and accurate patient note that contains relevant information regarding the history, physical examination, differential diagnosis, and diagnostic workup. This is a test that relies not so much on how much one studies and what one knows but how one does things. This book was written for those examinees who will be competent health providers in the future but, for now, need help preparing for this new kind of test experience.

This book will walk you through the USMLE Step 2 CS examination from beginning to end. The tips provided will give you the guidance and direction you need to do your best. The more than fifty practice cases will sharpen your skills in interviewing, physical examination, communication, and patient note writing preparing you for every possible interaction. Although licensure bureaus, medical schools, and disciplines may vary in small ways, the overall structure of the standardized patient examination will be the same as in this book. So read carefully and relax on the day of the examination. Having the right preparation and confidence for the Step 2 CS can make a challenging experience easy, educational, and fun.

Jo-Ann Reteguiz
June 2004

Acknowledgments

I wish to acknowledge the University of Medicine and Dentistry of New Jersey–New Jersey Medical School and, in particular, the Department of Medicine for its exceptional commitment to patient care and medical education.

REVIEWERS

Faculty Reviewers

Marilyn A. Miller, M.D.
ASSOCIATE CHIEF OF STAFF FOR
    EDUCATION
VETERANS ADMINISTRATION
    HEALTHCARE SYSTEM
EAST ORANGE, NEW JERSEY

Beverly R. Delaney, M.D.
DEPARTMENT OF PSYCHIATRY
VETERANS ADMINISTRATION
    HEALTHCARE SYSTEM
EAST ORANGE, NEW JERSEY

Saray Stancic, M.D.
CHIEF OF INFECTIOUS DISEASES
VA HUDSON VALLEY HEALTH CARE SYSTEM
MONTROSE, NEW YORK

Lawrence E. Harrison, M.D.
ASSISTANT PROFESSOR OF SURGERY
CHIEF, DIVISION OF SURGICAL ONCOLOGY
DEPARTMENT OF SURGERY
UNIVERSITY OF MEDICINE AND DENTISTRY
    OF NEW JERSEY–NEW JERSEY MEDICAL
    SCHOOL
NEWARK, NEW JERSEY

Arlene Bardeguez, M.D.
ASSOCIATE PROFESSOR OF OBSTETRICS
    AND GYNECOLOGY
DEPARTMENT OF OBSTETRICS AND
    GYNECOLOGY
UNIVERSITY OF MEDICINE AND DENTISTRY
    OF NEW JERSEY–NEW JERSEY MEDICAL
    SCHOOL
NEWARK, NEW JERSEY

Iris Ayala, M.D.
ASSISTANT PROFESSOR OF OBSTETRICS
    AND GYNECOLOGY
DEPARTMENT OF OBSTETRICS AND
    GYNECOLOGY
UNIVERSITY OF MEDICINE AND DENTISTRY
    OF NEW JERSEY–NEW JERSEY MEDICAL
    SCHOOL
NEWARK, NEW JERSEY

Ralph Pellecchia, M.D.
DIRECTOR OF FAMILY HEALTH SERVICES
DEPARTMENT OF OBSTETRICS AND
    GYNECOLOGY
JERSEY CITY MEDICAL CENTER
JERSEY CITY, NEW JERSEY

Norman Hymowitz, Ph.D.
PROFESSOR OF PSYCHIATRY
DEPARTMENT OF PSYCHIATRY
UNIVERSITY OF MEDICINE AND DENTISTRY
    OF NEW JERSEY–NEW JERSEY MEDICAL
    SCHOOL
NEWARK, NEW JERSEY

Resident and Student Reviewers

Paulo B. Pinho, M.D.
CHIEF MEDICAL RESIDENT 2003–2004
UNIVERSITY OF MEDICINE AND DENTISTRY
    OF NEW JERSEY–NEW JERSEY MEDICAL
    SCHOOL
NEWARK, NEW JERSEY

Vivek N. Dhruva, D.O.
CHIEF MEDICAL RESIDENT 2003–2004
UNIVERSITY OF MEDICINE AND DENTISTRY
    OF NEW JERSEY–NEW JERSEY MEDICAL
    SCHOOL
NEWARK, NEW JERSEY

Michael Demyen, M.D.
CHIEF MEDICAL RESIDENT 2004–2005
UNIVERSITY OF MEDICINE AND DENTISTRY
    OF NEW JERSEY–NEW JERSEY MEDICAL
    SCHOOL
NEWARK, NEW JERSEY

Rina Shah, M.D.
CHIEF MEDICAL RESIDENT 2004–2005
UNIVERSITY OF MEDICINE AND DENTISTRY
    OF NEW JERSEY–NEW JERSEY MEDICAL
    SCHOOL
NEWARK, NEW JERSEY

Lydia Estanislao, M.D.
RESIDENT, DEPARTMENT OF NEUROLOGY
UNIVERSITY OF MEDICINE AND DENTISTRY
    OF NEW JERSEY–NEW JERSEY MEDICAL
    SCHOOL
NEWARK, NEW JERSEY

William Sanchez, M.D.
UNIVERSITY OF MEDICINE AND DENTISTRY
    OF NEW JERSEY–NEW JERSEY MEDICAL
    SCHOOL
CLASS OF 1999
NEWARK, NEW JERSEY

Mastering the
USMLE
Step 2 CS
(Clinical Skills Examination)

Section A: The Examination

Introduction

Very much more time must be . . . given to those practical portions of the examinations which afford the only true test of . . . fitness to enter the profession. The day of the theoretical test is over.

SIR WILLIAM OSLER, 1885

WHAT IS THE STEP 2 CS?

The Step 2 CS (Clinical Skills Examination) is a standardized patient (SP) examination given to U.S., Canadian, and international medical students and graduates and is now a USMLE (U.S. Medical Licensing Examination) requirement for licensure. All graduates wishing to practice medicine in the United States are required to take this examination. The test consists of 10 to 12 stations or encounters (1 to 2 may be experimental stations and are not counted), each lasting 15 minutes. The test mirrors a physician in a clinic, office, emergency room, or hospital setting. Some of the most commonly tested complaints are headache, weakness, hypertension, asthma, impotence, dizziness, peptic ulcer disease, kidney stones, upper respiratory tract infections, and urinary tract infections.

At each station, you will encounter a different SP who is trained to accurately portray a real-life patient. You must ask the SP the appropriate questions to obtain the right history of present illness and then perform the accurate and focused physical examination. Throughout the history and physical examination, you are being graded on your interpersonal skills and proficiency in communication. After the interaction with the SP, you proceed to a 10-minute interstation (post-encounter station) to compose an accurate, organized, and legible written record of the encounter, called the *patient note*.

History taking and performance of a physical examination are considered data-gathering (DG) ability and are evaluated by the SP. The DG score is combined with the patient note score. The health care professional trained to read the patient note rates the note based on legibility, organization, and interpretation of the data (pertinent positives and negatives, differential diagnosis, and workup). The patient note score is automatically reduced if you suggest any dangerous action. The DG and the patient note scores are averaged over 10 stations, so if you perform poorly at one test station, you may be able to compensate by performing well at another. The DG and patient note scores are combined to form the final grade of the first component, called the *Integrated Clinical Encounter* (ICE), of the Step 2 CS.

The SP will evaluate your interpersonal/communication skills (IPS) and proficiency in the spoken English language (ENG). These are the second and third components of the Step 2 CS final grade. The IPS score is based on your interpersonal skills in interviewing (e.g., use of open-ended questions), giving information to the patient (e.g., counseling), how you interact with the patient (rapport), and your attitude during the interaction. The four IPS skills may be rated as unsatisfactory, marginally satisfactory, good, or excellent.

The ENG score is based on your grammar, pronunciation, and how difficult it is for the SP to understand you. The four ratings used for the ENG score are low, medium, high, and very high comprehensibility. An international graduate examinee who has taken the Test of Spoken English (TSE) and scored above 35 most likely will have no difficulty with the CSE ENG score component.

A below-average score on one of the three components of the Step 2 CS will result in a failure. Your overall score (pass or fail) will be reported to you within 8 weeks of your exam date, but delays in grade reporting are expected. Retake examinations are allowed 3 months after a failure.

The Step 2 CS is a multidisciplinary examination balancing the specialties of Internal Medicine, Surgery, Pediatrics, Obstetrics and Gynecology, Psychiatry, and Family Medicine. Expect to see cases in Cardiology, Pulmonary Medicine, Gastroenterology, and Urology (favorite Step 2 CS topics). There is a mix of subacute, acute, and chronic problems. It is given to candidates daily at Clinical Skills Evaluation Centers in Philadelphia, Pennsylvania; Atlanta, Georgia; Los Angeles, California; Chicago, Illinois; and Houston, Texas (September 2005) at a cost of approximately $1200. A comprehensive orientation manual and videotape providing practical and useful information about the examination are available at the USMLE website.

Who Is the Standardized (Simulated) Patient?

A standardized patient (SP) is a layperson who is trained to portray a specific clinical problem. An SP may be a healthy person or someone with a stable physical finding. It is important to remember that an SP is not an actor. The SP memorizes a script, like an actor, but his or her main task is to critique the performance of each examinee.

SPs are chosen because of their intelligence and attention to detail. They remain objective and do not volunteer any information to examinees. They may interrupt you while you are speaking or performing the physical examination, but this is done to distract you. SPs are focused on your performance from the moment you walk into the testing room until the time you leave.

SPs accurately portray the emotional or physical symptoms required for the test station. They are chosen for a particular interaction because of their understanding of the medical or ethical problem of the case. The roles played by SPs are diverse so as to challenge your ability to remain nonjudgmental and sensitive regardless of a patient's gender, race, intellect, sexual orientation, or ability to pay.

Just like a real patient, the SP will ask you specific questions about his or her presenting problem, e.g., "Tell me Doctor, does this mean I have cancer?" or "Doctor, am I having a heart attack?" The SP is challenging you with these questions, and they must not be ignored or avoided. Occasionally the SP will be a "difficult patient"; he or she will not be courteous or cooperative. You, however, must continue to extract the best possible history from the SP and remain calm. You must address the concerns of the SP as you would those of a real patient. If you do not know the answer to an SP's question, simply say you don't know.

All acceptable and unacceptable SP behavior and dialogue is memorized by the SP. Maneuvers necessary for an accurate physical examination, when required for a specific case, are rehearsed to perfection. You therefore should expect a remarkably realistic and experienced SP.

During each test station, the SP is evaluating you to assess whether the tasks on the checklist are being adequately carried out (checklists are covered in later chapters). Your nonverbal and verbal behavior is critically observed. Is the doctor arrogant? Is the doctor indifferent? Is the doctor interested in my problem? Does the doctor look bored? Is the doctor empathetic? Does the doctor seem aware of my modesty during the physical examination? Keep in mind that the main objective of the SP is to assess your ability to obtain a focused history and perform a physical examination while interacting effectively with him or her.

The Day of the Test

Prior to the start of the SP examination, you are given a detailed but brief orientation explaining how you go from station to station and your role at the patient note station. You always have sufficient time to travel from one place to another and read the instructions for the new test station, so never distress yourself or others by rushing.

The SP encounters take place in private rooms resembling a physician's office. You should wear a white coat and bring a stethoscope. The rooms are equipped with gloves and the medical instruments necessary for that specific test station. The SP will be dressed appropriately. Testing rooms are equipped with video cameras that are hidden, so as not to detract from the realism of the interaction. Do not waste time trying to look for the video cameras; just assume that they exist at every test station.

Alarms or verbal announcements are used to signal the start and the end of a test station. Extra time is not allowed, and SPs are instructed to stop the interaction upon hearing the "end of the station" signal. A warning signal, indicating when only a few minutes are left at a station, is used to help you pace yourself. When only a few minutes are left at a station, you must:

1. Complete any remaining tasks in the history or physical examination that are considered to be critical to the test station.

2. Begin to achieve adequate closure with the SP. Discuss the differential diagnosis and your plan with the SP. Make sure the SP understands your plan, including the tests you will be ordering, the medications you will be prescribing, the follow-up appointment and the prognosis.

The grade you receive for each interaction is based on the checklist completed by the SP after you leave the encounter and on your patient note, which is reviewed by a qualified individual. The overall grade reflects your ability to gather the appropriate data while communicating and interacting effectively with each SP.

The Day of the Test

Step 1

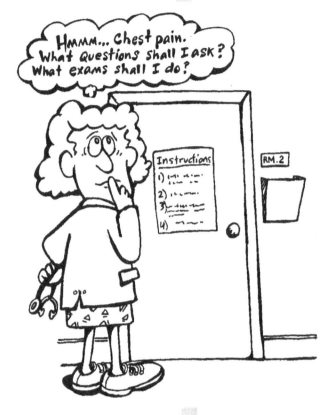

- Read "Instructions to the Examinee"
- Review the patient's name, chief complaint, and vital signs
- Formulate a mental checklist
- Knock on the door and enter
- Introduce yourself by name to the patient
- Address the patient by his or her last name (Mr./Mrs./Miss Smith)

Step 2

- Obtain a focused history (7 to 8 minutes)
- Do a relevant physical exam (4 to 5 minutes)
- Discuss your initial diagnostic impression and workup plan (1 to 2 minutes)
- Utilize your interpersonal skills
- 15-minute station

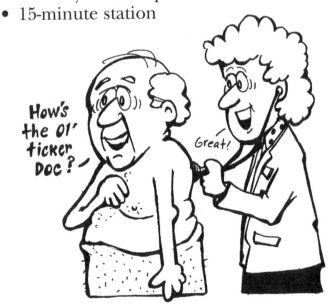

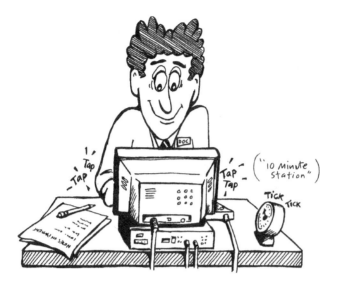

Step 3

The Step 2 CS Patient Note

- Write a pertinent history
- Describe the key physical findings
- List up to five possible diagnoses
- List up to five needed diagnostic tests/studies
- 10-minute station

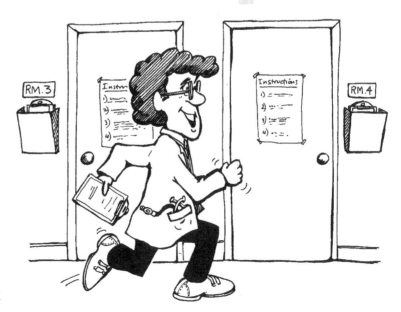

Step 4

- Proceed to the next patient

Beginning the Standardized Patient Encounter

A bad beginning makes a bad ending.

EURIPIDES

Instructions to the examinee are posted outside each examination room and must be read prior to starting a test station. You must read the instructions carefully. Important background information about the patient will be included in the instructions when relevant, such as age, past medical problems, and occupation.

The background information will help you prepare to perform the tasks to be evaluated at the test station. The instructions will inform you of the patient's chief complaint and reason for seeing the doctor (triage information). Vital signs will be included in the instructions if they are required for the station. The test center will provide you with scratch paper on which to write down pertinent information from the instructions if you so desire.

After you finish reading the instructions, you should consider the skills being tested and plan your patient interaction strategy. If you enter the test station prepared to begin, you will appear confident and knowledgeable, and an SP tends to remember a good first impression.

The instructions to the examinee will state what is required at each test station. Your tasks at each station are clearly stated, and you should not deviate from what is required. The instructions are covered with a sheet of paper, so do not uncover them until told to do so. There are instances when a patient complaint has nothing to do with the real reason the patient has come to the hospital or office. Drug-seeking patients, for example, might present complaining of severe migraine headaches or kidney stones. Sometimes the background information provided in the instructions to the examinee, if read carefully, will help expose these underlying problems.

Developing the Checklist

Where observation is concerned, chance favors only the prepared mind.

LOUIS PASTEUR

Each test station has specific objectives or checklist items reflecting the skills to be critically assessed by the SP. The SP will complete the checklist after you leave the room.

A checklist usually consists of 25 items and is restricted to the skills being tested at each test station. The checklist is actually the test and is never revealed to you. It consists of the tasks that must be accomplished successfully by you during an SP encounter. These checklist items may be in the areas of history, physical examination, or communication.

In order to perform well on the SP examination, you must learn how to mentally formulate the "hidden" checklist at the beginning of each test station. After obtaining the chief complaint for the SP, you should focus on the presenting problem and mentally decide which specific parts of the history of the present illness, past medical history, social history, family history, and physical examination are essential for the particular encounter.

Regardless of the task you are asked to perform at a test station, approach every SP as if he or she were a real patient, using your best bedside manner, because your communication skills are being assessed at each station. The SP's perception of you as a physician is vital to performing well.

Following is an example of a checklist for a test station:

1. The instructions given at the start of the test station reveal a chief complaint of abdominal pain in a 31-year-old man. His vital signs are normal except for a temperature of 101.0°F.

2. You are asked to obtain a history and perform a physical examination in 15 minutes.

3. Try to develop your own "mental checklist."

4. What is important for you to ask and do for this patient?

5. Check your "mental checklist" against the actual examination checklist.

6. Would you have passed this test station?

SP CHECKLIST FOR MR. SMITH

Responses by the imaginary SP appear in parentheses after each checklist item.

History of Present Illness. The Examinee Asked About:

___ 1. onset of pain ("4 hours ago.")

___ 2. location of pain ("Right lower side and around the navel.")

___ 3. quality of pain ("Deep and burning.")

___ 4. any aggravating factors ("Deep breath, movement, food.")

___ 5. any alleviating factors ("Lying still helps.")

___ 6. severity of pain ("On a scale of 1 to 10, where 10 is the worst, this is a 9.")

___ 7. any association with vomiting ("Two episodes at home.")

___ 8. any blood in the vomitus ("No.")

___ 9. any association with a change in bowel movements ("No diarrhea or constipation.")

___10. any blood in the stools ("No.")

___11. any urinary problems ("No.")

___12. any past medical problems ("No.")

___13. any medication use ("No.")

___14. any alcohol abuse ("No.")

___15. any allergies ("None.")

Physical Examination. The Examinee:

___16. listened for bowel sounds over all four quadrants (normal bowel sounds heard).

___17. palpated gently throughout my abdomen (patient has hyperesthesia over T11 and T12 dermatome).

___18. palpated deeply throughout my abdomen (pain localized to right lower side of abdomen).

___19. elicited rebound tenderness (severe pain when letting go of right lower abdomen).

___20. attempted to elicit a psoas or obturator sign (both are positive).

___21. checked for costovertebral angle tenderness (none).

Communication Skills. The Examinee:

___22. washed his or her hands before the start of the examination.

___23. introduced self warmly as he or she came into the room.

___24. seemed to care about my discomfort and pain.

___25. discussed the diagnostic possibilities with me (i.e., appendicitis, diverticulitis, kidney stones, pyelonephritis).

___26. put me at ease when I stated that my cousin nearly died when her appendix burst.

___27. discussed the diagnostic tests that would be done (blood work, urinalysis, radiographs).

___28. discussed initial management and plan (intravenous fluids, checking urine and blood-work results, observation, possible surgery).

___29. discussed prognosis (very good).

Approach to the SP

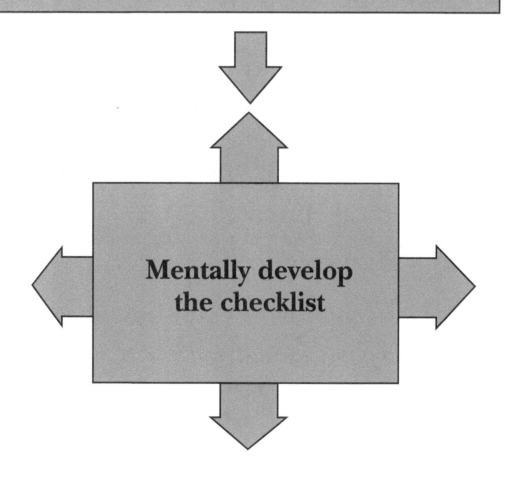

Read the
instructions to the examinee

Focus on the patient's problem

Mentally develop
the checklist

The Checklist Is Everything

Develop the following checklist items for each patient:

- History of Present Illness (Pertinent +/-)

- Past Medical History

- Family History/Social History

- Physical Examination (Pertinent +/-)

- Communication Skills

The History

Much unhappiness has come into the world because of bewilderment and things left unsaid.

FYODOR DOSTOYEVSKY

When you enter a test station, introduce yourself to the SP. Begin the interview with an open-ended question such as "How can I help you today?" or "What brings you to the hospital today?" Greet the patient warmly by shaking hands and smiling.

Start building upon the chief complaint given in the examinee instructions by eliciting accurate information in a logical and systematic fashion. For example, a common SP complaint is pain. An SP may have abdominal pain, chest pain, or a headache. You should ask the seven pertinent pain-related questions:

1. onset of pain
2. location of pain
3. quality of pain
4. severity of pain
5. alleviating factors
6. aggravating factors
7. associated symptoms

An examinee should probe into areas of the past medical history and family history when appropriate. If the social history is relevant, all the patient's habits should be investigated, including the use of tobacco, alcohol, illicit drugs, and caffeine. The patient's lifestyle including exercise habits, sexual history, diet, hobbies, travel, occupation, and environmental exposure to toxins (even radon) should be included if relevant to the chief complaint. Personal life problems and emotional stresses should be explored when necessary.

Try to use open-ended questions when possible and never repeat the same questions. Demonstrate appropriate listening skills, such as good eye contact and a leaning-forward posture at eye level. Be silent when necessary and try not to interrupt the patient when he or she is speaking. Nod your head once in a while to let the SP know you are listening.

You will want to be as thorough as possible and obtain a complete history at each test station, but you need to stay focused and within areas of appropriate questioning. Do not make a hasty diagnosis and end the interview prematurely. Consider the differential diagnosis for each presenting problem.

Make sure that you address the following four questions at each test station:

1. What organ system am I dealing with?
2. What are the likely causes of the problem?
3. What risk factors could have contributed to the problem?
4. What complications of the problem exist in this patient?

At the end of the interview, you must achieve closure by summarizing the patient problem, soliciting questions or concerns, and discussing the plan. Remember to say "thank you" and "good-bye" in an appreciative manner before leaving each test station.

The History

**Make sure you address the following
four questions at each test station:**

1. What **organ system** am I dealing with?
2. What are the **likely causes** of the problem?
3. What **risk factors** could have contributed to the problem?
4. What **complications** of the problem exist in this patient?

**To be systematic and ensure that all aspects of
the complaint of pain are covered, ask the
seven pain-related questions**

1. onset and chronology
2. location and radiation
3. quality of pain
4. severity of pain
5. alleviating factors
6. precipitating factors
7. associated symptoms

The Physical Examination

If you are directed to perform a physical examination, utilize the data you have gathered from the history to keep your physical examination focused on the chief complaint. The SP mentally critiques your physical examination skills and will judge whether you have performed the essential maneuvers and techniques appropriately. *This is a test not only of what you know and do but also of how you do it.*

Although the physical exam should be focused, you must always be thorough. For example, if an SP is portraying a college student with a sore throat and the history leads you to a diagnosis of mononucleosis, you should perform an abdominal exam, looking for hepatosplenomegaly, as well as a throat examination.

In real life, the SP may have the abnormal physical finding you elicit (e.g., a heart murmur, gallop, hepatomegaly, or splenomegaly) or simply may have been trained to imitate a particular finding (Murphy's sign, Kernig's sign). Some physical findings are simulated with make-up (jaundice). Explain to the patient what parts of the physical examination you are going to do before doing them ("I'm going to listen to your heart now.") and explain your findings ("Your heart sounds normal").

Be prepared to perform the following categories of the physical examination:

1. vital signs, including repeating blood pressure if pertinent (e.g., patient with hypertension) or orthostatic changes when necessary.

2. ears, eyes, nose, mouth, and neck examination, including proper use of an ophthalmoscope and otoscope; proper examination of the thyroid.

3. upper and lower extremity musculoskeletal examinations.

4. lung examination, including the use of proper sequence (inspection, palpation, percussion, auscultation) and listening anteriorly or at the right midaxillary line to auscultate the right middle lobe.

5. heart examination, including palpation of the point of maximum impulse; auscultation over all valve areas, and listening for radiation of murmurs when indicated; performing augmentation maneuvers, including the Valsalva maneuver and inspiration when indicated.

6. abdominal examination, including the use of proper sequence (inspection, auscultation over all quadrants, percussion of the liver at the midclavicular and midsternal

lines, and palpation); evaluating for splenomegaly by percussion or palpation; inspecting for Cullen's sign or Turner's sign; eliciting a Murphy's sign, obturator sign, or psoas sign; eliciting costovertebral angle tenderness if appropriate.

7. the Step 2 CS examination will not require a corneal reflex, breast, pelvic, rectal, or genital examination; these may be included in the patient note if appropriate as important diagnostic tests; you may, however, mention these to the patient verbally and explain why they are needed. If a corneal, rectal, breast, pelvic, or genital examination was done by the nurse practitioner (this will be stated in the instructions), don't forget to explain the results to the patient.

8. neurologic examination, including cranial nerves (I to XII), motor (tone and strength), sensory (position sense, touch, and vibration), and cerebellar (finger-nose-finger, heel-shin, and rapid alternating movements) examinations; assessing deep tendon reflexes; eliciting the Babinski sign; testing for a Romberg sign; eliciting Kernig's and Brudzinski's signs for meningitis.

9. mental status examination, including the use of a Mini-Mental State Examination or alcohol screening instrument when appropriate; level of depression; memory, insight, judgment, abstract reasoning, fund of knowledge, right/left orientation, writing ability, spatial ability, drawing ability, homicidal ideation, suicidal ideation, paranoid ideation, and hallucinations.

10. functional assessment of an elderly patient to document impairments such as vision loss, hearing loss, immobility, frailty, and gait disturbances.

Let the patient know when you are going to begin the physical examination. Wash your hands before every examination. Show consideration for the patient's discomfort and pain. If the patient exhibits signs of distress, acknowledge this and do what you can to make him or her more comfortable. Do not repeat painful maneuvers unless absolutely necessary. Keep the patient draped as much as possible during the examination and ask the patient for permission prior to touching him or her or removing any clothing. Use the examination table pull-out extension if you wish the patient to recline. Perform the examination in a logical sequence so the patient does not have to constantly change position. Tell the patient what you plan to do and explain findings when appropriate. Ask the patient to dress as soon as the physical examination is over and help the patient on and off the examination table. You should not begin a discussion with the patient if he or she is partially undressed.

The Physical Examination

Vital Signs	Blood pressure, pulse rate, respiratory rate, temperature, orthostatics (systolic blood pressure decreases by 20 mmHg, or diastolic blood pressure decreases by 10 mmHg, or heart rate increases by 20 beats per minute when patient stands from a supine position)
HEENT Exam	Funduscopic and otoscopic exams, thyroid palpation, jugular venous distention, carotid bruits
Pulmonary Exam	IPCA (inspection, palpation, percussion, auscultation), crackles, wheezes, egophony, pectoriloquy, tachypnea, Kussmaul and Cheyne-Stokes breathing
Cardiac Exam	PMI (point of maximum impulse—see p. 21), auscultation, augmentation maneuvers (e.g., Valsalva, inspiration), gallops, rubs, murmurs, lifts, heaves
Abdominal Exam	IAPP (inspection, auscultation, percussion, palpation), Cullen's, Turner's, Murphy's signs, obturator and psoas signs, costovertebral angle tenderness, splenomegaly, hepatomegaly, shifting dullness
Neurologic Exam	Cranial nerves, motor, sensory, cerebellar, DTRs (deep tendon reflexes), Babinski's, Romberg's, Kernig's, and Brudzinski's signs
Mental Status	Mini-Mental State Exam, CAGE screening for alcoholism, depression screening, memory, insight, judgment, abstract reasoning, fund of knowledge, right/left orientation, writing ability, spatial ability, drawing ability, homicidal ideation, suicidal ideation, paranoid ideation, and hallucinations.
Geriatric Functional Assessment	ADL (activities of daily living) and IADL (instrumental activities of daily living) assessment, vision loss, hearing loss, mobility and/ or gait disturbance, "get-up-and-go test"

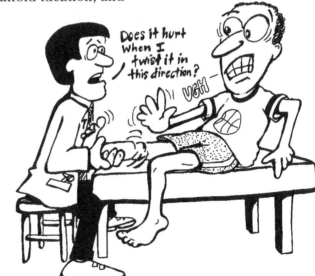

Don't repeat painful maneuvers.

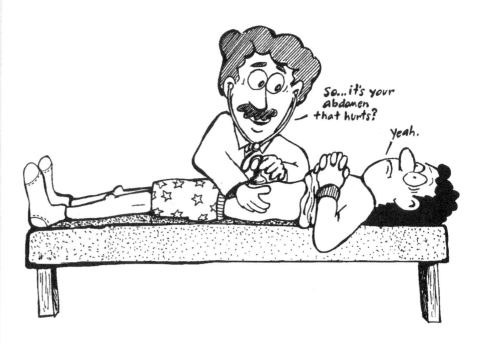

- Do not do a comprehensive physical examination
- Do a focused physical examination based on the presenting problem
- Perform maneuvers appropriately
- Don't repeat painful maneuvers
- Show consideration for the patient's discomfort

This is a test not only of what you know and do, but also of how you do it.

Physical Examination Findings That May Be Seen in an SP

HEENT
Hearing loss/visual loss
Ptosis

Cardiovascular System
Bruits (abdominal, carotid, renal, thyroid)
Chest pain—reproducible with palpation
Hypotension/hypertension (using a fake cuff)
Cuff that is either too small or too large for the patient
Tachycardia/bradycardia

Respiratory System
Airway obstruction
Cheyne-Stokes respirations
Cyanosis
Diminished breath sounds/pneumothorax
Hemoptysis
Hoarseness
Kussmaul respirations
Shortness of breath/dyspnea/tachypnea
Wheezing/stridor

Gastrointestinal System
Abdominal tenderness/rebound/guarding
Breath odor of diabetic ketoacidosis
Caput medusae/fetor hepaticus
Costovertebral angle tenderness
Cullen's sign/Turner's sign
Melena/hematochezia
Murphy's sign
Pregnancy
Psoas sign/obturator sign
Vomiting/hematemesis

Extremities
Casts for fractures
Deep venous thrombosis
Joint restriction/joint immobility
Joint warmth/joint erythema
Pretibial myxedema

Psychiatry
Anxiety/panic attack/hyperventilation
Anger/hostility
Dementia/delirium/depression
Hypomania/mania
Altered mental status/confusion

Neurologic System

Dilated pupil/nonreactive pupil
Alcohol intoxication/alcohol withdrawal
Aphasia
Ataxia/incoordination
Babinski's sign/extensor plantar reflex
Asterixis
Brudzinski's sign/Kernig's sign
Chorea
Coma/unresponsiveness
Decerebrate/decorticate rigidity
Dizziness/vertigo
"Doll's eye" response
Dysarthria
Facial nerve paralysis/Bell's palsy
Gait abnormalities
Hyperactive tendon reflexes/clonus
Muscle rigidity/cogwheel rigidity
Muscle spasms/spasticity
Muscle weakness
Nuchal rigidity
Photophobia
Romberg's sign
Seizures
Tinel's sign/Phalen's sign
Tremor

Skin

Anaphylaxis
Allergic reaction/hives
Bruising/ecchymosis/petechiae
Burns
Cellulitis
Diaphoresis/perspiration
Janeway lesions/Osler's nodes
Jaundice
Lyme disease rash/erythema chronicum migrans
Malar rash
Palmar erythema
Photosensitivity
Rashes
Skin track marks
Spider telangiectasia
Surgical scars
Tophi

Five Simple Steps to Effective Communication

Expect your communication skills to be assessed *continuously* during the SP examination. Certain stations may be devoted totally to communication, as when you are instructed to deliver bad news to a patient at a test station. At other stations, the SP will observe you throughout the history taking and, if required, the physical examination and then reflect on your effectiveness in overall communication, language proficiency, and use of interpersonal skills. These are essential tasks that, if not performed to the satisfaction of the SP, will result in a poor outcome for the test station. You will be proficient in communicating with patients by following these five simple steps:

1. **EXPLAIN YOUR FINDINGS**   You must make an effort to educate every patient about the chief complaint by clearly explaining the features of the disease or problem. You must explain the pertinent findings on physical examination and discuss the course you expect the problem to take. Try to identify the patient's emotional response and understanding of the problem; then offer your support and reassurance. Do not give the patient a premature diagnosis. **Always try to present a differential diagnosis.** If you are not sure what the diagnosis is, simply say so. Don't give the patient false information or false reassurance.

2. **DISCUSS THE PROGNOSIS**   The prognosis should be stated clearly even if the patient fails to bring this up. Reassure the patient when and if recovery may be expected. You should discuss available family and community support systems in the case of severe or terminal illness. Discuss the patient's feelings about the prognosis and help the patient cope if the prognosis is poor.

3. **OUTLINE THE PLAN**   You must counsel the patient regarding compliance and persuade him or her to undergo the necessary care. You should clearly outline the steps of care and check to see whether the patient is planning to cooperate with the plan. Discuss the patient's feelings regarding the plan. Make it clear to the patient that you will continue to participate in his or her care even when consultation is necessary.

4. **INVOLVE THE PATIENT IN THE PLAN** You must explain how the patient can assist in his or her own care (as by teaching a diabetic patient to check his or her own fingerstick or teaching an asthmatic patient to follow peak flowmeter readings). Lifestyle changes (safe sexual practices, diet, exercise) or risk-factor reduction (tobacco cessation, limiting sun exposure) requires the patient to commit to change. You must invite the patient to participate actively in his or her own management and plan.

5. **EDUCATE THE PATIENT** You must incorporate the principles of preventive health care and counsel the patient appropriately. Examinees should demonstrate fundamental knowledge of these measures during the SP examination.

Throughout the performance of the five communication tasks, you should use appropriate language and avoid medical terminology (jargon). Your approach to the patient should be organized and systematic. Because of time constraints, you must stay on track to meet all five of the communication test objectives, but transitions from one area to another should be hardly noticeable. Listen to the SP carefully and allow him or her to complete statements without interruption. If you must interrupt the patient, as in the case of a manic or overly talkative patient, do so tactfully.

Ralph Waldo Emerson said that "when the eyes say one thing and the tongue another, a practiced man relies on the language of the first." Therefore be flexible enough to follow up an SP's nonverbal clues by responding appropriately to the emotional situation. Do not continue to march through the communication tasks while ignoring the SP's emotional state. Stopping to address the emotion may not allow you enough time to complete all the communication tasks, but—in the long run—doing so will reflect positively on your overall performance. While exchanging information with the SP, always convey a sense of warmth and show empathy, concern, and consideration for the SP's feelings. Be sensitive to his or her pain and dignity.

Lack of good communication skills can be the downfall of an examinee, because these skills are evaluated at each test station. It is difficult to remember the principles of good communication when you are trying to be thorough and get the job done, especially with the overall time constraints, but failure to interact appropriately with the SP will have an adverse effect on your overall performance. In every encounter with an SP, always remember the five simple steps of effective communication:

E—Explain your findings

P—discuss the **P**rognosis

P—outline the **P**lan

I—Involve the patient in the plan

E—Educate the patient

Five Simple Steps
to Effective Communication

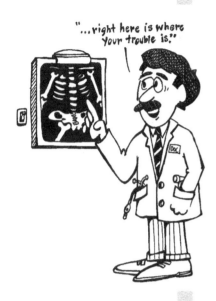

"...right here is where your trouble is."

E—**E**xplain your findings
- Features of the disease
- Pertinent physical exam findings
- Don't give a premature diagnosis

P—discuss the **P**rognosis
- Prognosis should be stated clearly
- Help the patient cope

P—outline the **P**lan
- Counsel the patient regarding compliance
- You and the patient are allies

I—**I**nvolve the patient in the plan
- Lifestyle changes
- Risk-factor reduction

E—**E**ducate the patient
- Preventive measures

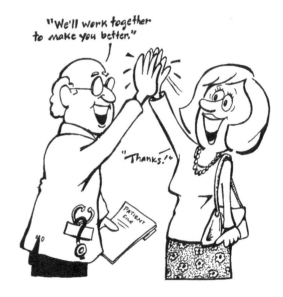

"We'll work together to make you better."

"Thanks!"

Preventive Measures to Discuss with the SP

1. Alcohol, drug, and tobacco counseling

2. Cancer screening

   • Breast self-examination, mammography, and Pap smear
   • Testicular and prostate examination
   • Fecal occult blood testing (FOBT)
   • Screening sigmoidoscopy/colonoscopy
   • Skin examination

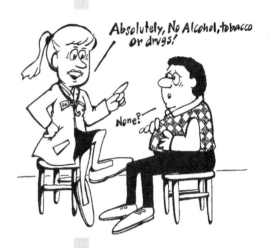

3. Infectious disease prevention

   • Annual purified protein derivative (PPD)
   • Safe sexual practices
   • Vaccinations [influenza, pneumococcal, hepatitis B, measles-mumps-rubella (MMR), diphtheria, tetanus]

4. Proper diet and exercise

   • Prevention of heart disease, diabetes, cancer, hypertension, and osteoporosis

5. Methods of stress reduction (when necessary)

6. Environmental and occupational hazards (when appropriate)

7. Injury prevention

   • Wearing automobile seat belts
   • Using bicycle helmets properly

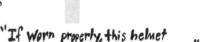

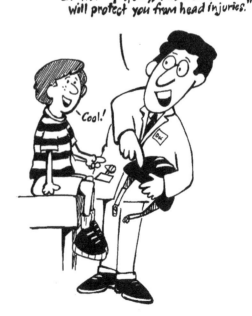

Improving Your Interpersonal Skills Quickly

HISTORY-TAKING SKILLS

- Use open-ended questions—e.g., "What is troubling you ?" "Can you tell me about your symptoms?"
- Use pauses; allow the patient time to think and react.
- Never interrupt the patient when he or she is speaking.
- Go smoothly from one area of discussion to another.
- Use listening techniques such as good eye contact and an open (arms uncrossed), leaning-forward posture at eye level.
- Repeat the last statements made by the SP so that he or she will continue speaking.
- Use plain, understandable language.
- Do not be in a rush; let the patient answer a question before you ask another question.
- Be open to questions; never avoid or ignore a question.
- Show interest in the patient's story; never act bored.

PHYSICAL EXAMINATION SKILLS

- Wash your hands in front of the patient.
- Do not examine the patient through the gown but keep the patient draped as much as possible.
- Ask the patient for permission prior to touching him or her or removing clothing.
- Tell the patient what you plan to do.
- Explain your physical examination findings.
- Be sensitive to the patient's pain, suffering, and discomfort.
- Never begin a discussion with the patient partially undressed.
- Never repeat painful maneuvers.
- Help the patient on and off the exam table.

COMMUNICATION AND INTERPERSONAL SKILLS

- Introduce yourself to the patient warmly; shake hands.
- Acknowledge the emotion the patient is showing, then discuss the emotion, e.g., "You seem sad."
- Don't give the patient more information than he or she can handle.
- Demonstrate empathy when appropriate.
- Demonstrate an attitude of confidence, reliability, and warmth.
- Seek the patient's point of view; inquire about any concerns the patient may have.
- Never be judgmental or confrontational with a difficult patient.
- Establish a partnership with the patient—e.g., "We'll work together to make you better."
- Do not give the patient false reassurance.
- Praise the patient—e.g., "You are coping very well with this illness."
- Provide the patient with closure.

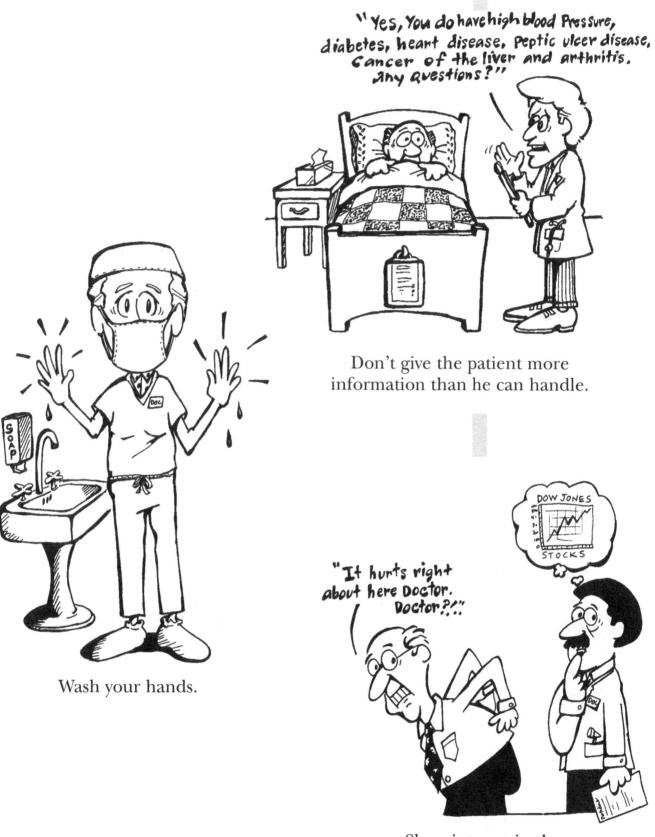

Don't give the patient more information than he can handle.

Wash your hands.

Show interest in the patient's story. Never act bored.

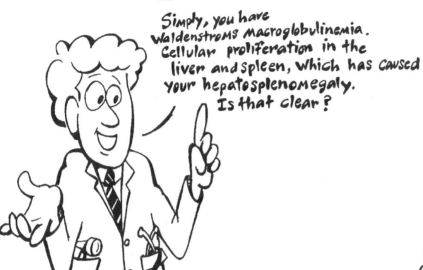

Use plain, understandable language.

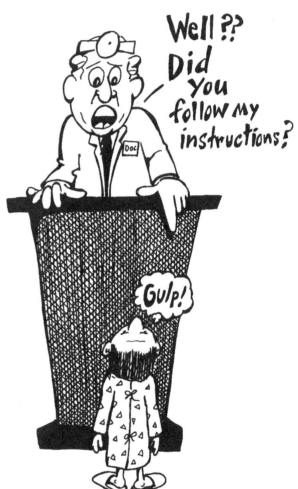

Never lecture the patient.

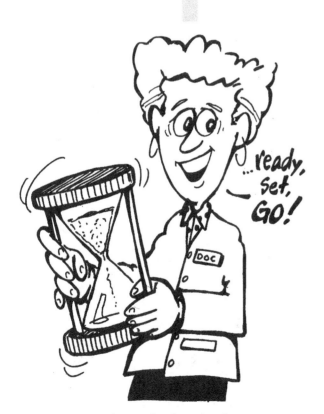

Don't rush the patient.

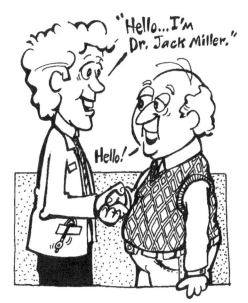

Introduce yourself.

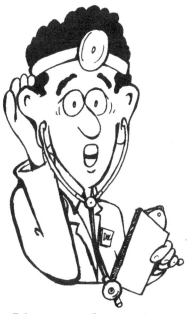

Listen to the patient.

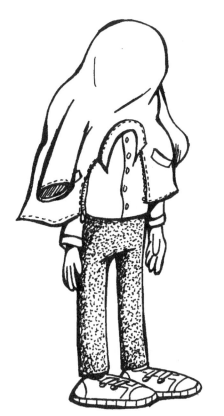

Don't embarrass
the patient.

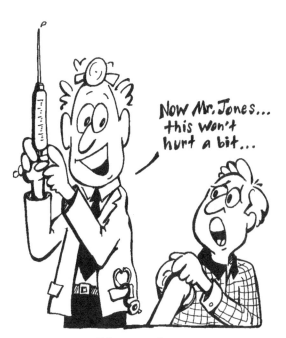

Never give
false reassurance.

Common Communication Challenges

It's either easy or impossible.

Salvador Dali

An examinee should be prepared to manage at least one difficult communication problem during an SP examination. Below are the more common communication challenges encountered during an SP examination.

1. **DELIVERING BAD NEWS TO A PATIENT**   This station may require you to discuss an abnormal mammogram report or an abnormal Pap smear result or to inform a patient that he or she has cancer, HIV/AIDS, or Alzheimer's disease. In these encounters, you must quickly establish good rapport and address the patient's specific needs and emotions. Try to summarize the problem and talk about the prognosis, but only if you feel that the patient can handle it. You must stop often and acknowledge the patient's distress. Inquire about the patient's thoughts and concerns. Talk about the patient's support system, such as family or close friends. Offer to help the patient inform loved ones about the medical condition. Give a step-by-step follow-up plan and offer your ongoing support. If the patient is able to discuss it, talk about a living will or an advance directive. Always inquire at the end of the interview: "Is there anything we didn't cover?"

2. **THE DECISION TO FORGO TREATMENT**   This test station may involve a patient who refuses a lifesaving blood transfusion due to religious beliefs; refuses surgery, intubation, or resuscitation; or requests removal of a life-sustaining device such as a ventilator or feeding tube. At this point you must inquire about the patient's emotional well-being to make sure that the patient is not depressed, confused, or angry. You must make sure that the patient understands the disease and the consequences of the decision (death). Ask whether family members or loved ones are aware of the patient's decision. When there is a substitute decision maker for the patient, make sure you are speaking to the appropriate person. Agree to honor the request and offer the patient support from a psychiatrist or member of the clergy. Let the patient know that the decision can be changed

in the future if he or she so desires. Ask about other life-sustaining treatments, such as oxygen or antibiotics. Describe your intentions to the patient clearly ("I will go to the chart and write the 'do not resuscitate' order."). This test station requires empathy and good closure.

3. **THE NEED TO TELL THE TRUTH**   The examinee is asked by a family member not to tell a patient about an illness. During this interaction, you should inquire about the reasons for the request and inform the family member that the patient has the right to know about the medical problem. Let the family member know that if the patient asks directly about his or her health, ethically, you must tell the truth. If the patient does not ask, you will not give the patient any information the family member feels the patient cannot handle. At this test station, you must never promise not to tell the patient.

4. **THE NONCOMPLIANT PATIENT**   These patients are usually misinformed about their disease and the reasons for the medications. You must make sure that the patient understands the illness and why the medications are being prescribed. Discuss the reasons for noncompliance with the patient and switch to an alternative medication if side effects are responsible. You must interest the patient in his or her own condition and enter into an agreement of compliance with the patient. Schedule follow-up visits and praise the patient's progress. If a patient prefers a nontraditional therapy, such as acupuncture or hypnosis, you must counsel the patient on the need for traditional therapy along with the alternative method. Respect the patient's right to individuality.

5. **THE BATTERED PATIENT**   This patient may present to the physician's office with a minor complaint. The astute examinee will obtain the history of violence during the interview or notice bruises on the patient. Regardless of the presenting complaint, if you notice bruises on any patient, ask specifically about violence in the home. Inform the patient that domestic violence is illegal and that police involvement helps prevent further abuse. Inquire about weapons in the home. In cases of spousal abuse, talk about the children and inform the patient that violence in the home affects the future behavior of children. Acknowledge to the wife that it is difficult to leave an abusive husband. Show concern for the safety of the patient and inquire about available support systems. Offer your own support, counseling, and follow-up. Be prepared to discuss domestic violence support systems in the community.

6. **THE ISSUE OF CONFIDENTIALITY**   A good example of this is an adolescent requesting contraception who does not wish her parents to know. First, you must discuss the benefits and risks of contraception with the adolescent. If you feel that the adolescent patient has the competence and judgment of an adult, you can prescribe contraception and not share the information with the parents. If the parents wish to know why their daughter visited the physician, you must clearly inform the parents of their daughter's right to confidentiality. Try to convince the parents to discuss the issue directly with their daughter. Offer to counsel the family together as a way of improving communication. Keep in mind that the parent-physician relationship is as confidential as the daughter-physician relationship. You must not divulge information about the parents' visit to the daughter.

7. **THE OVERTALKATIVE PATIENT**   The talkative, hypomanic, or manic patient is very difficult to interrupt, but you must do so tactfully without sacrificing rapport. With this kind of patient, it is often better to use the closed-ended style of questioning. As difficult as it may seem, since the patient will not let you get a word in edgewise, try to remain in control of the interview. Avoid becoming frustrated, angry, and impatient. Focus on obtaining an accurate history and physical examination.

8. **THE ALCOHOLIC PATIENT**   You must identify this issue during routine history taking and physical examination. The patient may complain of tremors, insomnia, blackouts, frequent falls, weight loss, sexual dysfunction, depression, or problems with personal relationships. The patient may smell intoxicated or appear intoxicated during the interview. You must address the alcohol abuse in a nonjudgmental and nonconfrontational manner. Inquire as to why the patient drinks. Ask about the frequency and quantity of the patient's alcohol consumption. Ask about a family history of alcoholism. Inquire about attempts to stop drinking made in the past. Ask about stresses in the patient's life that may be contributing to the drinking and the relapses. Identify the patient in denial. When necessary, integrate the **CAGE** questionnaire into the interview ("Have you ever attempted to **C**ut down on your drinking?, Have people **A**nnoyed you by criticizing your drinking?, Have you felt **G**uilty about your drinking?, Do you need an **E**ye-opener first thing in the morning to cure a hangover or steady your nerves?"). Tell the patient you have confidence in his or her ability to stop drinking. Ask the patient if

he or she is willing to work on the problem; then discuss specific treatment options (support groups, hospitalization for withdrawal, outpatient counseling, medications). Negotiate a plan and offer your continued understanding and support.

9. **THE SUBSTANCE-ADDICTED PATIENT**   In treating a drug abuser, including the drug-seeking patient, you must control your own biases and remain respectful. Try to appear comfortable discussing the drug use and initiate the topic if you notice track marks on the patient's skin. Inquire about the pattern of use and explore the concerns the patient may have about stopping. Discuss the health risks of drug use. Inquire about the patient's support system and develop a clear plan of management for the drug problem. Offer the patient choices for detoxification (hospitalization, outpatient management) and state clearly that you will treat withdrawal symptoms. Discuss follow-up visits to assess progress and to reinforce the patient's efforts.

10. **THE SMOKER**   You must inquire about nicotine addiction, whether it be cigarette smoking, exposure to passive smoke, or use of smokeless tobacco. On physical examination, if you observe nicotine stains on the patient's fingernails, bring up the topic of smoking cessation. Ask about the number of years the patient has been smoking and the number of cigarettes smoked per day. Ask how many times the patient tried to quit smoking and explore the reasons for relapse. Educate the patient about nicotine as a risk factor for coronary artery disease, cancer, and lung disease. Ask the patient specifically whether he or she is willing to stop. Show the patient that you have confidence in his or her ability to stop ("You can do it!"). Discuss the strategies to quit smoking (gum, patch, pills, behavior modification). Negotiate a plan with the patient and discuss follow-up for monitoring progress. Remember to give the "stop smoking" message to every patient who smokes.

11. **THE PATIENT WITH SPECIAL EMOTIONAL PROBLEMS** This category is broad and diverse and includes the hostile patient ("I'm going to sue you.") and the anxious patient ("This headache is so bad that I'm sure I have a brain tumor."). These patients still require a thorough interview and, if appropriate, a focused physical examination. These patients need a great deal of patience, empathy, and reassurance. Offer understanding and do your best to address the patient's concerns.

12. **THE PATIENT NEEDING CONSENT FOR A PROCEDURE**   You must obtain informed consent by explaining step by step how the procedure is performed. Explain the purpose of the procedure and the possible complications. Explain the indications, contraindications, risks, and benefits of the procedure using plain and concise language. Tell the patient what his or her experience during the procedure will be and assure the patient that his or her comfort during the procedure will be a priority. Respect the a patient's decision to refuse a procedure. You should be prepared to obtain informed consent for arterial line placement, arthrocentesis, autopsy, organ donation, bronchoscopy, placement of a central venous line catheter, flexible sigmoidoscopy or colonoscopy, liver biopsy, lumbar puncture, abdominal paracentesis, placement of a Swan-Ganz catheter, HIV testing, and thoracentesis.

COMMON COMMUNICATION CHALLENGES

Delivering bad news to a patient	• Abnormal mammogram or Pap smear • Positive HIV test • Recently diagnosed cancer or Alzheimer's disease
The patient who decides to forego treatment	• Patient refuses lifesaving surgery, blood transfusion, intubation, resuscitation, or feeding • Family member requests removal of life support
The patient's right to be informed	• The patient has the right to know the truth about his or her disease and its prognosis
The noncompliant patient	• Make sure the patient understands the illness and the need for medication • Interest the patient in his or her condition and discuss the reasons for noncompliance
The battered patient	• Carefully obtain a history of violence; note bruises or evidence of trauma
The patient's right to confidentiality	• Respect the confidentiality of the patient–physician relationship
The overtalkative patient	• In the manic or hypomanic patient, tactfully interrupt and use closed-ended style of questioning • Avoid becoming impatient or frustrated
The alcoholic patient	• Address the alcohol abuse issue in a nonjudgmental and nonconfrontational manner • Integrate the CAGE questionnaire into the interview
The substance-addicted patient	• Offer detoxification choices • State that you will treat withdrawal symptoms • Control your own biases
The smoker	• Discuss strategies to quit smoking
The patient with special emotional problems	• The hostile or anxious patient • Address the patient's concerns
Obtaining informed consent	• Explain the indication, risks, benefits, and possible complications using plain and concise language

The Step 2 CS Patient Note: How to Pass the Written Part

NOTE

This note must contain the pertinent positives and negatives (relating to the presenting problem) obtained during the history-taking, including relevant information about the past medical history, social history, family history, and review of systems. The pertinent positives and negatives found on the physical examination must also be discussed in the patient note. You are then asked to list up to five diagnostic possibilities and up to five immediate diagnostic studies you would order. The CS patient note interstation does not require any further test interpretation. You are not required to discuss treatment. The patient note should be an organized, logical, and legible note containing accurate information regarding the patient's history, physical examination, differential diagnosis, and diagnostic workup.

REVIEW OF SYSTEMS:
PERTINENT POSITIVES AND NEGATIVES

The Step 2 CS challenges an examinee's ability to obtain a thorough history and formulate a broad differential diagnosis. The review of systems is an essential component of the CS examination and must be thorough and relevant. The examinee must be able to justify the differential diagnosis and list the pertinent positives and negatives for each presenting problem. A Step 2 CS examinee should memorize the review of systems and practice writing the patient note, using pertinent negatives and positives. **For the Step 2 CS, think in terms of the organ system involved, not the disease or your diagnosis**.

General	weight loss, weight gain, fatigue, chills, night sweats, overall general health
Skin	rashes, lumps, itchiness, dryness, hair changes, nail changes
Head	headaches
Eyes	double vision, blurred vision, eye redness, eye discharge, watery eyes, light bothers eyes (photophobia), wears reading glasses, history of glaucoma or cataracts
Ears	hearing loss, ringing in ears (tinnitus), room spinning (vertigo), dizziness, infections, discharge
Nose	history of allergies and hay fever, frequent colds, nasal congestion, nosebleeds, sinus problems
Mouth/Throat	hoarseness, bleeding gums, mouth sores, bad teeth, sore tongue, taste disturbance, sore throat, trouble swallowing
Neck	neck swelling (lymphadenopathy or goiter)
Breasts	nipple discharge, nipple inversion, bleeding nipple, asymmetry of the breasts, lumps, tender breasts, monthly self-examination, last mammogram
Respiratory	cough, chest pain, wheezing, shortness of breath, dyspnea on exertion, bloody cough, history of tuberculosis, pneumonia, asthma, last purified protein derivative (PPD) test, last chest x-ray
Cardiac	chest pain, pressure or tightness, palpitations, wakes up short of breath (paroxysmal nocturnal dyspnea), number of pillows slept on (orthopnea), shortness of breath, dyspnea on exertion, fainting, dizziness, swelling of feet, history of angina, myocardial infarction, congestive heart failure, hypertension, high cholesterol level
Gastrointestinal	abdominal pain, indigestion, loss of appetite, food intolerance, difficulty swallowing, painful swallowing, nausea, vomiting, coffee-ground emesis, constipation, diarrhea, blood or mucus in stools, blood in vomitus, change in bowel movements, jaundice, dark-colored urine, tarry stools, history of gallstones, pancreatitis, hepatitis, ulcer, and hemorrhoids

Urologic	painful or frequent urination; blood in urine; cloudy urine; wakes up at night to urinate (nocturia); trouble starting, holding, or stopping urine; history of urinary tract infection or stones
Genital (F)	menarche, last menstrual period, number of pregnancies, miscarriages or abortions, menopause, hot flashes, vaginal discharge, vaginal itching, abnormal vaginal bleeding, menstrual cramps, change in menstrual pattern, history of sexually transmitted diseases, painful intercourse, last Pap smear
Genital (M)	discharge from penis, sores on penis, painful or swollen testicles, history of hernias, history of sexually transmitted diseases, problems with erections, impotence
Rheumatologic	back pain, joint pain, swollen joints, warm joints, joint deformities, muscle weakness, history of gout, osteoarthritis, or rheumatoid arthritis
Peripheral Vascular	varicose veins, leg swelling, leg cramps, cold hands and feet, phlebitis, leg pain with walking (claudication)
Neurologic	headache, dizziness, weakness, numbness, fainting spells, problems with walking or coordination, room spinning (vertigo), tremors, problems with memory, problems with controlling urination (incontinence), history of seizures, paralysis, or strokes
Psychiatric	sadness, crying, irritability, nervousness, anxiety, fearfulness, hopelessness, sexual troubles, sleep disturbances, depression, hearing voices, thoughts about suicide, history of mental illness
Hematologic	bruises, pallor, history of anemia or blood transfusions
Endocrinologic	excessive urination, hunger or thirst, tremors, weight change, fatigue, feeling hot or cold all the time (temperature intolerance), history of thyroid disease or diabetes mellitus

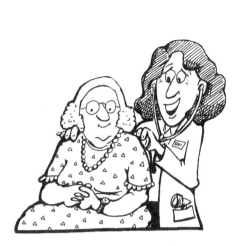

Medicine

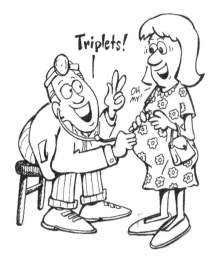

Obstetrics & Gynecology

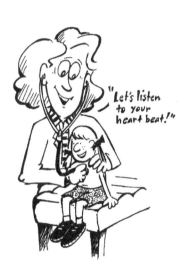

Pediatrics

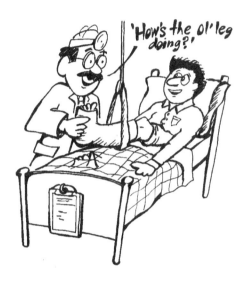

Surgery

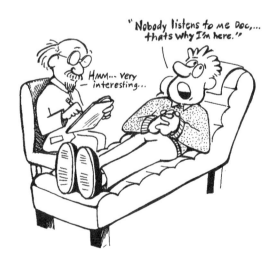

Psychiatry

Section B: Practice Cases: Mastering the Checklist and Patient Note

General Case Instructions

The cases that follow are examples of actual Step 2 CS (Clinical Skills Examination) cases. Read the instructions given at the beginning of each case and quickly develop your own checklist. Ask the SP whatever you think is pertinent, perform the appropriate physical examination if required, develop a differential diagnosis and plan, then check your strategy and checklist-developing ability against the actual SP checklist. Complete each checklist within 15 minutes and aim for a score of at least 70 percent. Then try to write your patient note in less than 10 minutes. You must write a relevant history, physical examination, differential diagnosis, and diagnostic workup.

Remember, it is the SP who is grading your checklist performance. The history you obtain, the physical examination you perform, and the way you communicate must match up with the SP's checklist for a passing grade. Remember, it is a health professional (usually a resident physician) who is reviewing your note, so it must be organized, logical, and medically correct. List pertinent parts of the history of present illness, past medical history, review of systems, social history, and family history. Keep in mind, however, that not every one of these categories will necessarily be pertinent to every case. Include pertinent positive and negative findings from the physical examination when applicable. Consider a range of possible diagnoses and list them in order of likelihood. Write your immediate plans for the diagnostic workup. Include a rectal, pelvic, breast, and genital exam if pertinent. Select fundamental tests (do not request an MRI scan for every patient). Do not request thyroid studies or a thyroid panel (order TSH and T_4 tests specifically). Do not order a chemistry panel (be more specific) or a liver profile (order an AST, ALT, etc.). You can, however, order component tests, such as a CBC, urinalysis, arterial blood gas, and electrolytes. Do not include any plans for management, such as hospitalization, medication, or consultation. Match your completed patient note with the patient note example. Remember, you must complete your patient note in 10 minutes or less.

To help you during the simulation, the responses of the SP during the examination are in parentheses at the end of each checklist item. Review the learning objectives provided to enhance your understanding of the medical problem. A good understanding of the case will allow you to write a clear, organized, and accurate patient note. Pearls in history-taking, physical examination, and patient note writing are included, when appropriate, to help you prepare for future cases.

Good Luck Examinee!

PRESENTING PROBLEMS

1. 70-year-old woman with forgetfulness
2. 46-year-old woman complaining of fatigue and weight gain
3. 65-year-old woman complaining of hearing loss
4. 20-year-old woman complaining of a cough for 4 days
5. 25-year-old man complaining of a sore throat
6. 68-year-old man requesting pain medications
7. 50-year-old woman requesting a blood pressure check
8. 55-year-old man complaining of chronic abdominal pain
9. 48-year-old man with chest pain
10. 25-year-old woman with leg pain
11. 35-year-old man with a chronic cough
12. 73-year-old woman with arm and leg weakness
13. 25-year-old female with a rash
14. 65-year-old man with difficulty swallowing
15. 62-year-old man with a history of frequent falls
16. 18-year-old man with a headache
17. 18-year-old woman with burning on urination
18. 18-year-old man with a rash
19. 20-year-old woman with rectal bleeding
20. 41-year-old man with blurred vision
21. 70-year-old man with difficulty urinating
22. 63-year-old woman who has become withdrawn
23. 40-year-old man with abdominal pain
24. 30-year-old man with a rash
25. 31-year-old woman with a wrist injury after a fall
26. 50-year-old woman with hand tingling
27. 33-year-old man with back pain
28. 17-year-old with shortness of breath
29. 31-year-old with difficulty "catching breath"
30. 4-month-old for well-baby visit
31. 19-year-old with urethral discharge
32. 59-year-old with 6-week history of shortness of breath
33. 19-month-old with new seizure
34. 26-year-old with lower abdominal pain
35. 50-year-old woman with hot flashes
36. 22-year-old woman with abdominal pain

37. 24-year-old pregnant woman with vaginal bleeding
38. 30-year-old woman with worsened menstrual cramps
39. 25-year-old pregnant woman for prenatal visit
40. 37-year-old woman with third-trimester bleeding
41. 20-year-old girl with weight loss
42. 45-year-old man despondent since the death of his wife
43. 26-year-old woman with frequent chest pain
44. 32-year-old woman emotionally drained since giving birth
45. 50-year-old man with insomnia
46. 52-year-old woman with abdominal pain
47. 35-year-old man with left-sided back pain
48. 50-year-old man with diffuse abdominal pain
49. 77-year-old man with left lower abdominal pain
50. 32-year-old man hit in the stomach with a baseball bat

Case 1

Please evaluate Mrs. Doe, a 70-year-old retired schoolteacher. She is visiting her daughter, who is your longtime patient. Mrs. Doe's daughter feels that her mother has become forgetful over the last 2 years and she wants you to evaluate her.

Vital Signs:

Temperature	98.6°F
Blood pressure	129/81 mmHg
Heart rate	86 beats per minute
Respiratory rate	14 breaths per minute

Examinee's Tasks

1. Obtain a focused and relevant history.
2. Perform a focused and relevant physical examination.
3. Perform a functional status examination.
4. Discuss your initial diagnostic impressions with the patient.
5. Discuss follow-up tests with the patient.
6. After seeing the patient, complete paperwork relevant to the case.

Try to develop the checklist for this encounter based on the presenting problem. Use the next page to make your own checklist.

MY CHECKLIST

History of Present Illness. The Examinee:

1. _____
   _____
2. _____
3. _____
4. _____
5. _____
6. _____
7. _____
8. _____
9. _____
10. _____
    _____
    _____
11. _____
12. _____
    _____
    _____

Physical Examination. The Examinee:

13. _____
14. _____
15. _____
16. _____
17. _____
18. _____
19. _____
    _____
    _____
20. _____

Communication Skills. The Examinee:

21. _____
22. _____
23. _____
24. _____
25. _____
26. _____
27. _____

SP CHECKLIST FOR MRS. DOE

History of Present Illness. The Examinee:

___ 1.   started with an open-ended question, i.e., "What brings you in today?" ("My daughter insisted I come in, but I've never felt better.")

___ 2.   asked about past medical history, i.e., high blood pressure, heart attack, stroke, irregular heartbeat ("No.")

___ 3.   asked about any use of medications ("None.")

___ 4.   asked about alcohol use ("None.")

___ 5.   asked about changes in weight ("No.")

___ 6.   asked about any history of falls or head trauma ("None.")

___ 7.   asked if I was having trouble remembering things ("No.")

___ 8.   asked about neurologic symptoms, i.e., weakness, dizziness, gait problems, incontinence ("No.")

___ 9.   asked about home living arrangements ("I live with two cats.")

___10.   asked about loneliness or sadness ("My husband died 10 years ago; I play bingo at the church every Tuesday; I teach reading at the community center; I visit the sick at the hospital after church on Sundays; I play bridge with my friends; I think my life is rich and full.")

___11.   asked about support systems ("My daughter is always there for me and I have supportive girlfriends.")

___12.   asked about at least three instrumental activities of daily living, i.e., shopping, cooking, money management, housework, telephone use, and travel outside the home ("I did take the wrong bus a few times, my house is a mess, I let my neighbor shop for me, my phone was disconnected because I did not pay the bill, I stopped cooking when the stove caught fire and I did forget to pay my rent 3 months in a row, but that's normal for people my age, isn't it?")

Physical Examination. The Examinee:

___13.   checked my orientation to person, place and time (orientation normal)

___14.   felt over my thyroid gland (gland is normal in size and consistency)

___15.   listened to both sides of my neck with stethoscope (no carotid bruits heard).

___16.   tested my strength in both arms and legs (normal strength in arms and legs).

___17.   tested my sensation in arms and legs, i.e., touch, vibration or moving my big toe up or down (normal sensation)

___18.   tested reflexes in arms and legs (normal reflexes).

___19.   conducted parts of the Mini-Mental State Examination (MMSE), i.e., checked for at least three of the following: spell "world" backwards, serial sevens, three-object recall, follow three-stage command, copy design (patient could not calculate, spell backwards, recall objects, copy design, or follow three-stage command).

___20.   asked me to walk across the room to check my gait (normal gait).

Communications Skills. The Examinee:

___21.   greeted me warmly.

___22.   had an organized approach to gathering information.

___23.   discussed the diagnostic possibilities with me (i.e., Alzheimer's disease, multi-infarct dementia, hypothyroidism).

___24.   inquired about my understanding of the problem.

___25.   gave a follow-up plan [blood work, computed tomography (CT) scan of the head].

___26.   asked for permission to speak with my daughter to discuss the problem.

___27.   offered partnership and ongoing support throughout my illness.

If you performed 19 of these 27 tasks, you passed this test station.

You have 10 minutes to complete your patient note.

HISTORY—Include significant positives and negatives from the history of present illness, past medical history, review of systems, and social and family history.

_____

_____

_____

_____

_____

_____

_____

_____

_____

_____

_____

PHYSICAL EXAMINATION—Indicate only the pertinent positive and negative findings related to the patient's chief complaint.

_____

_____

_____

_____

_____

_____

_____

_____

_____

_____

DIFFERENTIAL DIAGNOSIS—In order of likelihood, write no more than five differential diagnoses for this patient's current problems.

1. _____

2. _____

3. _____

4. _____

5. _____

DIAGNOSTIC WORKUP—Immediate plans for no more than five diagnostic studies.

1. _____

2. _____

3. _____

4. _____

5. _____

A SATISFACTORY PATIENT NOTE

HISTORY—Include significant positives and negatives from the history of present illness, past medical history, review of systems, and social and family history.

The patient is a 70-year-old former schoolteacher with no significant past medical history who is referred by her daughter for a 2-year history of "forgetfulness." Mrs. Doe, however, has no complaints and feels that she is not becoming forgetful. She denies weight change, dizziness, weakness, incontinence, or gait problems. She takes no medications and does not smoke cigarettes or drink alcohol. She denies recent falls or head trauma. Since her husband's death 10 years ago, Mrs. Doe lives alone with her two cats. She has several girl-friends and spends her days volunteering in various church and community center activities. Although the patient is able to adequately perform her activities of daily living, she does have difficulty with her instrumental activities of daily living, namely, transportation, food preparation, and accounting.

PHYSICAL EXAMINATION—Indicate only the pertinent positive and negative findings related to the patient's chief complaint.

Vital signs are normal. The patient is pleasant, cooperative and in NAD. Grooming and hygiene are adequate.
HEENT: No evidence of head trauma, PERLA, EOMI. Fundi benign. Thyroid gland is normal in size and consistency; no carotid bruits.
Heart: Normal S_1 and S_2; no murmurs, rubs, or gallops.
Lungs: Clear to auscultation and percussion.
Abdomen: Positive BS, no tenderness or masses.
Musculoskeletal: Normal gait.
Neuro: Alert, oriented to person, place, and time.
   CN: II–XII intact
   Motor: Normal tone and strength
   Sensory: Normal position sense and vibration
   Cerebellar: Normal heel-shin, and finger-nose-finger
   DTR: 2+ diffusely
MMSE: Unable to recall three objects and could not perform serial sevens or spell "world" backwards.

DIFFERENTIAL DIAGNOSIS
In order of likelihood, write no more than five differential diagnoses for this patient's current problems.

1. Alzheimer's disease
2. multi-infarct dementia
3. hypothyroidism
4. vitamin B_{12} deficiency
5. depression

DIAGNOSTIC WORKUP
Immediate plans for no more than five diagnostic studies.

1. CT scan of the head
2. TSH level
3. vitamin B_{12} level
4. electrolytes
5. CBC

LEARNING OBJECTIVE FOR MRS. DOE
THE ASSESSMENT OF COGNITIVE IMPAIRMENT IN AN ELDERLY PATIENT

This 70-year-old woman has had a gradual worsening of cognitive function involving memory and judgment over the last several years. She is no longer independent in her instrumental activities of daily living and performed poorly on the MMSE.

Mrs. Doe uses no medications or alcohol that might explain her cognitive impairment. A subdural hematoma without a history of head trauma or fall is unlikely. There is no weight gain, bradycardia, or depressive symptoms to suggest hypothyroidism. Lack of depressive symptoms makes the diagnosis of pseudodementia unlikely as well. Normal-pressure hydrocephalus is often accompanied by gait apraxia and urinary incontinence, but the patient denied having these symptoms.

The normal cardiac, carotid artery, and neurologic examinations and the absence of vascular risk factors such as hypertension, heart disease, and a previous history of stroke make Alzheimer's disease the most likely etiology of dementia in this patient.

A physician should investigate the home situation and existing support system for every patient with dementia and offer interdisciplinary assistance from medical and community resources when necessary.

History-Taking Pearl: Know the Katz activities of daily living or ADLs (**DEATH** = **D**ressing, **E**ating, **A**mbulating, **T**oileting, **H**ygiene) and the instrumental activities of daily living or IADLs (**SHAFT** = **S**hopping, **H**ousekeeping, **A**ccounting, **F**ood preparation, **T**ransportation).

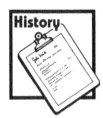

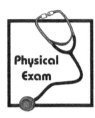

Physical Examination Pearl: A score of 23 out of a possible score of 30 on the Folstein MMSE indicates dementia. Other ways of testing a patient's functional mental status is to look for a concrete response to an interpretation of a proverb (e.g., "People in glass houses shouldn't throw stones" or "Don't cry over spilled milk") and by asking the patient to draw a clock face and indicate the time on it.

Familiarize yourself with the "get up and go" test to assess gait (the patient gets out of the chair, walks 10 ft, and returns to the chair). This test should be performed by the patient in less than 15 seconds.

Patient Note Pearl: The differential diagnosis for dementia includes Alzheimer's disease, multi-infarct dementia, normal-pressure hydrocephalus, hypothyroidism, vitamin B_{12} deficiency, folic acid deficiency, depression, neurosyphilis, and subdural hematoma. The **workup** for dementia includes complete blood count, electrolytes (especially calcium and renal function), liver function tests (hepatic encephalopathy), thyroid-stimulating hormone (TSH) level, syphilis serology, and vitamin B_{12} level. Certain patients may require other studies, such as HIV testing, folic acid level, erythrocyte sedimentation rate, CT scan of the head, electroencephalogram, and lumbar puncture.

NOTES

Case 2

Please evaluate Ms. Olive Goode, a 46-year-old woman who is complaining of fatigue and a 30-lb weight gain occurring over several months. She has been your private patient for nearly 20 years, with a history of hypertension controlled with oral hydrochlorothiazide 25 mg/day.

Vital Signs:

Temperature	98.8°F
Blood pressure	130/85 mmHg
Heart rate	52 beats per minute
Respiratory rate	14 breaths per minute

Examinee's Tasks

1. Obtain a focused and relevant history.
2. Perform a focused and relevant physical examination.
3. Discuss your initial diagnostic impressions with the patient.
4. Discuss follow-up tests with the patient.
5. After seeing the patient, complete paperwork relevant to the case.

MY CHECKLIST

History of Present Illness. The Examinee:

1. _____
   _____
2. _____
   _____
   _____
3. _____
4. _____
5. _____
6. _____
7. _____
8. _____
9. _____
10. _____
11. _____
    _____

Physical Examination. The Examinee:

12. _____
13. _____
14. _____
15. _____

Communication Skills. The Examinee:

16. _____
17. _____
18. _____
19. _____
20. _____
21. _____
22. _____
23. _____

SP CHECKLIST FOR MS. GOODE

History of Present Illness. The Examinee:

___ 1. started with an open-ended question, i.e., "What brings you in today?" ("Doctor, I have gained over 25 pounds in the last 2 months and I'm not even eating anything.")

___ 2. asked about depression, i.e., sadness, hopelessness, no interest in activities, inability to concentrate, loss of sexual desire ("I am feeling sad and hopeless lately; I have difficulty concentrating when I am balancing my checkbook and have no interest in activities or sex with my husband.")

___ 3. asked about the fatigue ("I'm tired all day; I have no energy; I really don't feel like myself.")

___ 4. asked about sleep habits ("I could sleep 20 hours a day if I didn't have to work.")

___ 5. asked about constipation ("Yes, I move my bowels once a week; I was never like that.")

___ 6. asked about cold intolerance ("I'm wearing a sweater even in hot weather; I am always cold.")

___ 7. asked about voice changes ("Yes; I feel like I'm hoarse.")

___ 8. asked about dry skin ("Yes; my skin is flaking off because of dryness.")

___ 9. asked about hair falling out ("Yes, it is falling out in clumps.")

___10. asked about a change in menses ("Yes, my periods are heavier than usual and last longer.")

___11. asked about a family history of thyroid disease ("My younger sister has a thyroid problem and takes pills for it; is that what I have?")

Physical Examination. The Examinee:

___12. looked in my mouth to check the size of my tongue (tongue slightly enlarged).

___13. examined my thyroid gland properly (gland normal and nontender).

___14. listened to my heart in at least three places (normal examination).

___15. examined the reflexes in my arms and legs (delayed relaxation phase in reflexes in arms and legs).

Communication Skills. The Examinee:

___16. had an organized approach to gathering information.

___17. used appropriate body posture.

___18. responded to my nonverbal clues.

___19. acknowledged my distress.

___20. discussed the diagnostic possibilities with me (i.e., hypothyroidism, Cushing's disease, depression).

___21. provided me with a plan (bloodwork, electrocardiogram, perhaps medication).

___22. inquired about my understanding of the plan.

___23. discussed the prognosis with me.

If you performed 17 of these 23 tasks, you passed this test station.

You have 10 minutes to complete your patient note.

HISTORY—Include significant positives and negatives from the history of present illness, past medical history, review of systems, and social and family history.

_____

_____

_____

_____

_____

_____

_____

_____

_____

PHYSICAL EXAMINATION—Indicate only the pertinent positive and negative findings related to the patient's chief complaint.

_____

_____

_____

_____

_____

_____

_____

_____

_____

_____

DIFFERENTIAL DIAGNOSIS—In order of likelihood, write no more than five differential diagnoses for this patient's current problems.

1. _____

2. _____

3. _____

4. _____

5. _____

DIAGNOSTIC WORKUP—Immediate plans for no more than five diagnostic studies.

1. _____

2. _____

3. _____

4. _____

5. _____

A SATISFACTORY PATIENT NOTE

HISTORY—Include significant positives and negatives from the history of present illness, past medical history, review of systems, and social and family history.

The patient is a 46-year old woman who complains of gaining 25 pounds over a 2-month period without an increase in appetite or food intake. She feels fatigued and seems to be sleeping more (20 hours a day sometimes). Recently, Mrs. Goode has feelings of sadness and hopelessness and has little interest in social activities, including a lack of sexual desire. She has trouble concentrating, especially when trying to balance her checkbook. The patient has a history of hypertension and takes HCTZ 25 mg daily. She does not use alcohol or drugs and does not smoke cigarettes. Family history is significant for a younger sister with thyroid disease who requires daily medications. Review of systems is remarkable for constipation, cold intolerance, dry skin, hair loss, and hoarseness.

PHYSICAL EXAMINATION—Indicate only the pertinent positive and negative findings related to the patient's chief complaint.

Patient is obese and appears exhausted. Speech is hoarse.
Vital signs are significant for bradycardia.
Skin: Dry and flaky. Missing lateral one-third of eyebrows. Hair on scalp is coarse. Fingers are puffy.
HEENT: Tongue is slightly enlarged. Thyroid nonpalpable.
Heart, lungs, and abdomen: Normal.
Neuro: Normal strength. Reflexes present but significant for delayed relaxation phase.

DIFFERENTIAL DIAGNOSIS
In order of likelihood, write no more than five differential diagnoses for this patient's current problems.

1. hypothyroidism
2. depression
3. Cushing's disease
4. chronic fatigue syndrome
5.

DIAGNOSTIC WORKUP
Immediate plans for no more than five diagnostic studies.

1. TSH level
2. T_4 level
3. CBC
4. electrolytes
5. electrocardiogram

LEARNING OBJECTIVE FOR MS. GOODE
DEALING WITH A NONSPECIFIC COMPLAINT
SUCH AS FATIGUE OR WEIGHT CHANGE

Thyroid problems must be considered in the differential diagnosis of any patient presenting with fatigue and an unexplained weight change. Ms. Goode is a 46-year-old patient who presents with three clinical features of hypothyroidism, namely, weight gain, fatigue, and bradycardia. With further questioning, the patient admits to having other common features of hypothyroidism, such as cold intolerance, dry, flaky skin, voice change, constipation, heavy and prolonged menses, and generalized hair loss. Patients with hypothyroidism may present with symptoms of depression, and Ms. Goode admits to feeling sad and hopeless.

A cardiac examination and electrocardiogram should be performed to verify the bradycardia and to look for signs of pericardial effusion. An examination of the mouth in a hypothyroid patient may reveal a thickened tongue. Deep tendon reflexes, especially those of the Achilles tendon, should be examined for a prolongation of the relaxation phase seen in a hypothyroid patient. Proper examination of the thyroid gland may reveal a nonpalpable thyroid gland or a nontender goiter.

The symptoms of hypothyroidism are insidious and erroneously attributed to normal aging. The examinee must be aware of the atypical and subtle presentation of this disease and order a test of the TSH level. Undiagnosed and untreated, hypothyroidism may progress to respiratory depression and coma.

History-Taking Pearl: Fatigue or lethargy ("feeling tired") is a common chief complaint. The **possible etiologies** include depression, hypothyroidism, acute diseases (infectious mononucleosis), and chronic diseases such as congestive heart failure, anemia, HIV, cancer, tuberculosis, and chronic fatigue syndrome. Medications (beta blockers and antihistamines) may also cause fatigue.

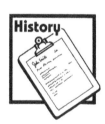

Patient Note Pearl: The **differential diagnosis** for weight gain includes hypothyroidism, depression, obesity, Cushing's disease, and anasarca (due to cardiomyopathy, nephrotic syndrome, and cirrhosis). The **workup** for hypothyroidism includes TSH, T_4, complete blood count (CBC), electrolytes, and cholesterol level. Anemia, hypercholesterolemia, hyponatremia, and an elevated creatine phosphokinase (CPK) level are often seen in hypothyroid patients. Serum triiodothyronine(T$_3$) is a poor test for primary hypothyroidism. It is not clinically useful to distinguish between the two major causes of hypothyroidism, Hashimoto's disease and chronic autoimmune thyroiditis (both have antibodies to thyroglobin and thyroid peroxidase and both are treated with hormone replacement therapy). Remember that amiodarone, used in treating certain cardiac arrhythmias, and lithium may cause hypothyroidism and should be included as a possible etiology when indicated.

NOTES

Case 3

A 65-year-old woman, Mrs. Edna West, is concerned about her hearing and has made an appointment to see you. Lately, she finds herself asking her husband to repeat things because she does not hear him well the first time he says them. Two days ago she went to the movies and had trouble hearing the dialogue.

Vital Signs:

Temperature	98.6°F
Blood pressure	120/80 mmHg
Heart rate	84 beats per minute
Respiratory rate	14 breaths per minute

Examinee's Tasks

1. Obtain a focused and relevant history.
2. Perform a focused and relevant physical examination.
3. Discuss your initial diagnostic impressions with the patient.
4. Discuss follow-up tests with the patient.
5. After seeing the patient, complete paperwork relevant to the case.

MY CHECKLIST

History of Present Illness. The Examinee:

1. _____
2. _____
3. _____
4. _____
5. _____
6. _____
7. _____
8. _____
9. _____
   _____
10. _____
11. _____
12. _____

Physical Examination. The Examinee:

13. _____
    _____
14. _____
15. _____
16. _____
    _____

Communication Skills. The Examinee:

17. _____
    _____
18. _____
19. _____
20. _____
21. _____
22. _____
23. _____

SP CHECKLIST FOR MRS. WEST

History of Present Illness. The Examinee:

___ 1. asked about the onset of the hearing loss ("It started gradually 6 months ago.")

___ 2. asked if one ear or both ears were affected ("It seems to be only the left ear.")

___ 3. asked if hearing loss was complete or partial in the affected ear ("Oh, I do hear something but not much.")

___ 4. asked about a history of vertigo ("No.")

___ 5. asked about a history of tinnitus ("No.")

___ 6. asked about ear discharge ("None.")

___ 7. asked about ear pain ("None.")

___ 8. asked about any history of trauma to the ear ("No.")

___ 9. asked about exposure to loud noises for extended periods of time, i.e., in the armed forces or due to occupation ("No; I was never in the armed forces and I work as a seamstress.")

___10. asked about any ear infections ("None.")

___11. asked about the use of any medications that may be ototoxic, i.e., diuretics, antibiotics ("None.")

___12. asked about a family history of hearing loss ("Yes, my mother wears hearing aids.")

Physical Examination. The Examinee:

___13. tested my hearing by covering each ear separately and whispering or rubbing fingers or by watch ticking (SP cannot hear in left ear).

___14   looked into both ears properly with otoscope (normal examination).

___15. performed the Weber test properly (SP will state that the stimulus is perceived on the right side).

___16. performed the Rinne test properly (SP will state that both air and bone conduction are decreased in left ear but air conduction is still greater than bone conduction).

Communication Skills. The Examinee:

___17. discussed the diagnostic possibilities for hearing loss with me (i.e., normal aging, noise exposure, previous infection).

___18. gently informed me that I needed a full audiologic evaluation.

___19. offered to schedule the audiology appointment for me.

___20. stated that I would benefit from an amplification device (hearing aid).

___21. did not cause me discomfort when examining me with the otoscope.

___22. was empathetic toward me.

___23. addressed my concerns about looking old with a hearing amplification device.

If you performed 17 of these 23 tasks, you passed this test station.

You have 10 minutes to complete your patient note.

HISTORY—Include significant positives and negatives from the history of present illness, past medical history, review of systems, and social and family history.

_____
_____
_____
_____
_____
_____
_____
_____
_____
_____

PHYSICAL EXAMINATION—Indicate only the pertinent positive and negative findings related to the patient's chief complaint.

_____
_____
_____
_____
_____
_____
_____
_____
_____
_____

DIFFERENTIAL DIAGNOSIS—In order of likelihood, write no more than five differential diagnoses for this patient's current problems.

1. _____
2. _____
3. _____
4. _____
5. _____

DIAGNOSTIC WORKUP—Immediate plans for no more than five diagnostic studies.

1. _____
2. _____
3. _____
4. _____
5. _____

A SATISFACTORY PATIENT NOTE

HISTORY—Include significant positives and negatives from the history of present illness, past medical history, review of systems, and social and family history.

Mrs. West is a 65-year-old seamstress who presents with a partial left-sided hearing loss that has progressively worsened over the last 6 months. She is having difficulty hearing her husband when he speaks to her and recently could not hear the dialogue at the movie theater. She denies tinnitus, vertigo, ear pain, or discharge. She did not suffer from ear infections as a child. She has never been exposed to loud noises and denies any history of trauma to the ear. She has never taken any medications that may have contributed to her hearing loss. She does not smoke or drink and eats a healthy diet. She tries to exercise regularly by taking long walks at least three times a week. Her family history is significant for hearing loss in her mother, who wears hearing aids.

PHYSICAL EXAMINATION—Indicate only the pertinent positive and negative findings related to the patient's chief complaint.

Patient appears anxious over hearing loss but is otherwise in NAD.
Vital signs are normal. Patient cannot perceive spoken voice in left ear.
HEENT: Left ear examination reveals no cerumen or foreign body. Tympanic membrane is normal. No perforation or sclerosis is evident. Cannot hear whisper or rubbed fingers when left ear is checked. Right ear is normal.
Weber test: Lateralizes to the right side.
Rinne test: Air and bone conduction are decreased in left ear but air conduction remains greater than bone conduction.
Heart, lungs, and abdomen: Normal.

DIFFERENTIAL DIAGNOSIS
In order of likelihood, write no more than five differential diagnoses for this patient's current problems.

1. sensorineural hearing loss
2. presbycusis
3. familial hearing loss
4.
5.

DIAGNOSTIC WORKUP
Immediate plans for no more than five diagnostic studies.

1. audiometry
2.
3.
4.
5.

LEARNING OBJECTIVE FOR MRS. WEST
THE PROPER ASSESSMENT OF HEARING LOSS

Approximately 50 percent of people over 65 years of age are hearing-impaired. A loss of hearing can occur from lesions in the external auditory canal or middle ear, causing a conductive hearing loss. Examples of conductive hearing loss include impaction due to cerumen, otitis externa, foreign body in the external canal, and tympanic membrane perforation.

Lesions of the inner ear or eighth cranial nerve cause a sensorineural hearing loss. When sensory hearing loss is suspected, the examinee must inquire about a history of infection, intense exposure to noise, and use of ototoxic drugs. Aging (presbycusis) may also cause sensory hearing loss. Neural hearing loss is due mainly to trauma, vascular events, an infectious process, and tumors such as acoustic neuroma.

The Rinne and Weber tuning fork tests are used to differentiate between conductive and sensorineural hearing losses. In conductive hearing loss, the Weber test lateralizes and the tone is perceived in the affected ear. The Weber test in a patient with a sensorineural hearing loss, as in the case of Mrs. West, results in the tone being perceived in the unaffected ear.

The Rinne test further helps to differentiate between a conductive and a sensorineural hearing loss. In conductive hearing loss, bone-conduction stimuli are perceived to be louder than air-conduction stimuli, while in sensorineural hearing loss, both air and bone conduction are diminished but air-conduction stimuli remain greater.

Mrs. West complains of gradual deterioration of her hearing. She has no vertigo or tinnitus, which are seen with tumors such as acoustic neuroma. Her otoscopic examination was unremarkable. She has no obvious risk factors to explain the hearing loss, such as trauma, noise exposure, infections, or medication use. She does, however, have a family history of hearing loss and a preexisting congenital abnormality may explain her recent deficit.

The Weber and Rinne examinations confirm a sensorineural hearing loss in this patient. An audioscope, if available, would have been the best instrument for accurately assessing the patient's hearing loss. The patient would benefit from a full audiologic evaluation followed by the fitting of an amplification device.

Physical Examination Pearl: Check for hearing loss by turning your face away from the patient and speaking. Practice the Rinne and Weber tests described above.

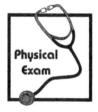

Physical Exam

Patient Note Pearl: In adults, the **differential diagnosis for conductive hearing loss** includes cerumen impaction, otitis externa, foreign body in the external canal, and tympanic membrane perforation. The **differential diagnosis for sensory hearing loss** includes aging, infection, noise exposure, and medication use. The **differential diagnosis for neural hearing loss** includes infection, trauma, a vascular event, and tumor. You should review the differential diagnosis for hearing loss in children.

Sensorineural hearing loss may be:
  congenital
    TORCH (toxoplasmosis, rubella, cytomegalovirus, herpesvirus) infections
    chromosomal abnormalities (trisomy 18, 21)
    syndromes (Alport's, Usher's)
    anatomic (aplasia of the cochlea)
  acquired
    bacterial infections (meningitis, otitis)
    viral infections (mumps, cytomegalovirus, herpesvirus, rubeola)
    vascular insufficiency (sickle cell disease, diabetes)
    trauma (noise, temporal bone fracture)
    tumor (leukemia, acoustic neuroma, neurofibromatosis)
    autoimmune, hypothyroidism, hypoparathyroidism
Conductive hearing loss may be due to:
    impacted cerumen, a foreign body, or otitis with effusion

NOTES

Case 4

Ms. Hazel Harris is a 20-year-old woman who presents to your office complaining of a cough.

Vital Signs:

Temperature	101.4°F
Blood pressure	120/75 mmHg
Heart rate	106 beats per minute
Respiratory rate	22 breaths per minute

Examinee's Tasks

1. Obtain a focused and relevant history.
2. Perform a focused and relevant physical examination.
3. Discuss your initial diagnostic impressions with the patient.
4. Discuss follow-up tests with the patient.
5. After seeing the patient, complete paperwork relevant to the case.

MY CHECKLIST

History of Present Illness. The Examinee:

1. _____
2. _____
3. _____
4. _____
5. _____
6. _____
7. _____
8. _____
9. _____
10. _____
11. _____
12. _____
13. _____
14. _____
15. _____
16. _____
17. _____
18. _____

Physical Examination. The Examinee:

19. _____
20. _____
21. _____
22. _____
23. _____
24. _____
25. _____
_____

Communication Skills. The Examinee:

26. _____
27. _____
28. _____
29. _____
30. _____

SP CHECKLIST FOR MS. HARRIS

History of Present Illness. The Examinee:

___ 1.   asked about the onset of cough ("Started 4 days ago.")

___ 2.   asked about production of sputum ("Small amount of thick green phlegm.")

___ 3.   asked about blood in the sputum ("No.")

___ 4.   asked about sore throat ("Maybe a little.")

___ 5.   asked about fever ("For the last 2 days, my temperature has been 101.5°F.")

___ 6.   asked about shaking chills ("Yes, I did have some chills last night.")

___ 7.   asked about night sweats ("None.")

___ 8.   asked about shortness of breath ("No.")

___ 9.   asked about pleuritic chest pain ("None.")

___10.   asked about past medical history ("None.")

___11.   asked about tobacco use ("I've been meaning to stop smoking; I've smoked 10 cigarettes a day for 3 years.")

___12.   asked about alcohol use ("None.")

___13.   asked about illicit drug use ("No.")

___14.   asked about contacts being ill ("Yes; everyone at work seems to have this bug, whatever it is.")

___15.   asked about occupation ("I work as a cashier in a toy store.")

___16.   asked about pets or animal exposure ("No.")

___17.   asked about any recent travel ("No.")

___18.   asked about last PPD placement ("2 years ago for employment purposes and it was negative.")

Physical Examination. The Examinee:

___19.   palpated throughout neck for swollen glands (none)

___20.   looked in throat (no erythema or exudate)

___21.   palpated over maxillary sinuses (no tenderness)

___22.   asked me to say "99" as moved hand from side to side over my back

___23.   tapped on my back from side to side

___24.   listened to front and back of my chest with a stethoscope

___25.   asked me to whisper or say the letter "e" while listening with a stethoscope (positive "e" to "a" changes and positive whispered pectoriloquy at the right base).

Communication Skills. The Examinee:

___26.   explained the results of the physical examination to me (consistent with pneumonia).

___27.   explained the diagnostic possibilities to me (i.e., pneumonia, tuberculosis, asthma).

___28.   explained the workup (chest radiograph).

___28.   explained the treatment (antibiotics, acetaminophen).

___29.   scheduled a follow-up appointment with me.

___30.   discussed tobacco cessation with me.

If you performed 21 of these 30 tasks, you passed this test station.

You have 10 minutes to complete your patient note.

HISTORY—Include significant positives and negatives from the history of present illness, past medical history, review of systems, and social and family history.

_____

_____

_____

_____

_____

_____

_____

_____

_____

_____

PHYSICAL EXAMINATION—Indicate only the pertinent positive and negative findings related to the patient's chief complaint.

_____

_____

_____

_____

_____

_____

_____

_____

_____

_____

_____

DIFFERENTIAL DIAGNOSIS—In order of likelihood, write no more than five differential diagnoses for this patient's current problems.

1. _____

2. _____

3. _____

4. _____

5. _____

DIAGNOSTIC WORKUP—Immediate plans for no more than five diagnostic studies.

1. _____

2. _____

3. _____

4. _____

5. _____

A SATISFACTORY PATIENT NOTE

HISTORY—Include significant positives and negatives from the history of present illness, past medical history, review of systems, and social and family history.

Ms. Hazel Harris is a 20-year-old woman who presents with a 4-day history of cough productive of thick, green-colored sputum. At home, she recorded a temperature of 101.5°F, which was accompanied by shaking chills and a mild sore throat. She denies chest pain, shortness of breath, night sweats, and hemoptysis. She has no past medical history and does not drink alcohol or use illicit drugs. She smokes approximately 10 cigarettes per day for over 3 years. She is interested in stopping smoking. She is employed as a cashier in a toy store and states that coworkers have had similar complaints. She has no recent travel and has no pets. A PPD was placed 2 years ago as a preemployment prerequisite and was nonreactive.

PHYSICAL EXAMINATION—Indicate only the pertinent positive and negative findings related to the patient's chief complaint.

Patient is well developed and well nourished. She is coughing every few minutes and is in mild respiratory distress.
T = 101.4°F. HR = 106 beats/min. RR = 22 breaths/min.
HEENT: No cervical lymphadenopathy. Throat without erythema or exudate. Maxillary sinuses nontender.
Lungs: Normal fremitus and dullness. Pectoriloquy and egophony at right base.
Heart and abdomen: Normal.
Extremities: No cyanosis or clubbing.

DIFFERENTIAL DIAGNOSIS
In order of likelihood, write no more than five differential diagnoses for this patient's current problems.

1. pneumonia
2. bronchitis
3. tuberculosis
4. asthma
5. tobacco addiction

DIAGNOSTIC WORKUP
Immediate plans for no more than five diagnostic studies.

1. chest x-ray
2. CBC
3. repeat PPD
4. sputum Gram's stain
5. pulse oximetry reading for oxygen saturation

LEARNING OBJECTIVE FOR MS. HARRIS
APPROACH TO THE PATIENT WITH AN ACUTE COUGH

Pneumonia is a common medical problem. The acute features of this disease include cough, production of purulent sputum, fever, and pleuritic chest pain. Patients usually complain of an upper respiratory tract infection prior to the onset of the more prominent features.

Streptococcus pneumoniae is the most common pathogen causing community-acquired pneumonia. Other pathogens responsible for pneumonia include viruses, *Haemophilus influenzae,* and, less commonly, *Mycobacterium tuberculosis.*

Atypical pneumonia is due primarily to *Mycoplasma pneumoniae.* The presentation is one of gradual onset of symptoms, dry cough, and extrapulmonary involvement. Other causes of atypical pneumonia include *Chlamydia pneumoniae* and *Legionella pneumophila.*

When suspecting pneumonia, a physician should inquire about risk factors that predispose an individual to aspiration, such as loss of consciousness from drug or alcohol use. The past medical history should document any existing comorbid conditions, such as diabetes mellitus and kidney, heart, or lung disease. A thorough social history including recent travel, hobbies, occupational history, animal exposure, and contact with ill individuals should be investigated.

On physical examination, the patient who presents with tachypnea, hypotension, or tachycardia requires hospitalization. Other indications for inpatient management of community-acquired pneumonia include age over 65 years, comorbid illness, leukopenia, and hypoxemia.

A thorough lung examination should include an evaluation for signs of consolidation, which may include increased tactile fremitus, dullness to percussion, and auscultation findings, such as crackles, bronchial breath sounds, egophony, and pectoriloquy.

A chest radiograph is critical to making the diagnosis of pneumonia, but the pattern of infiltration is not diagnostic for any specific organism. Bacterial pneumonia, however, is often a lobar infiltrate with air bronchograms and perhaps a pleural effusion, while viral and atypical pneumonias are usually diffuse or multilobar in distribution and rarely accompanied by an effusion.

Physicians treating an outpatient for a community-acquired pneumonia must form a partnership with the patient to ensure compliance with medications and follow-up visits. Any patient not responding appropriately to oral antibiotic therapy requires inpatient management.

Patient Note Pearl: The **differential diagnosis** for cough includes pneumonia, tuberculosis, asthma, bronchitis, congestive heart failure, and drug allergy. The **workup** includes a CBC and a chest radiograph. When indicated, other tests may include measurement of peak flow, sputum for acid-fast bacilli, oxygen saturation, and arterial blood gases. **Always discuss smoking cessation with every tobacco-using patient; discuss nicotine gum, nicotine patches, and behavioral therapy.**

Case 5

You are about to see Mr. Donald Dearborn, a 25-year-old college student, who presents to your office complaining of a sore throat.

Vital Signs:

Temperature	101.2°F
Blood pressure	115/75 mmHg
Heart rate	88 beats per minute
Respiratory rate	14 breaths per minute

You walk into the examination room and see a jaundiced young man in no acute distress.

Examinee's Tasks

1. Obtain a focused and relevant history.
2. Perform a focused and relevant physical examination.
3. Discuss your initial diagnostic impressions with the patient.
4. Discuss follow-up tests with the patient.
5. After seeing the patient, complete paperwork relevant to the case.

MY CHECKLIST

History of Present Illness. The Examinee:

1. _____
2. _____
3. _____
4. _____
5. _____
6. _____
7. _____
8. _____
9. _____
10. _____
    _____
11. _____
12. _____
13. _____
14. _____
    _____
15. _____
16. _____
    _____
17. _____

Physical Examination. The Examinee:

18. _____
19. _____
20. _____
21. _____
22. _____

Communication Skills. The Examinee:

23. _____
24. _____
25. _____
26. _____
27. _____
28. _____

SP CHECKLIST FOR MR. DEARBORN

History of Present Illness. The Examinee:

___ 1. asked about the onset or duration of sore throat ("I've had it for 7 days now.")

___ 2. asked about fever ("Yes, but never greater than 101.5°F.")

___ 3. asked about cough ("No.")

___ 4. asked about swollen glands ("Yes. I feel my neck glands are swollen and tender.")

___ 5. asked about the jaundice ("I noticed it yesterday for the first time.")

___ 6. asked about abdominal pain ("My upper abdomen feels swollen to me; no pain felt.")

___ 7. asked about nausea or vomiting ("None.")

___ 8. asked about loss of appetite ("Definitely yes. I just don't feel like eating anything at all.")

___ 9. asked about change in bowel movements ("No.")

___10. asked about past medical history ("No history of jaundice, hepatitis, blood transfusions, body piercing, or tattoos.")

___11. asked about medications ("None.")

___12. asked about illicit drug use ("No.")

___13. asked about alcohol use ("None.")

___14. asked about any risk factors for hepatitis A, i.e., eating shellfish, overcrowding, contaminated water or food ("No.")

___15. asked about ill contacts ("My girlfriend has a sore throat, fever, and swollen glands and is jaundiced too.")

___16. asked about sexual history ("I am heterosexual; one girlfriend; always use condoms now and with two previous partners.")

___17. asked about immunization against hepatitis B ("I did get that before starting college.")

Physical Examination. The Examinee:

___18. looked inside my mouth to examine throat (pharynx is erythematous).

___19. palpated my neck glands (neck is tender to palpation).

___20. tapped my liver to determine size.

___21. pressed over my abdomen (SP will complain of tenderness on right upper side).

___22. pressed over spleen area (SP will complain of tenderness on left upper side).

Communication Skills. The Examinee:

___23. washed hands before beginning physical examination.

___24. explained results of the physical examination (inflamed throat, swollen glands, tender liver).

___25. explained the diagnostic possibilities to me (i.e., mononucleosis, hepatitis A, B, or C).

___26. explained plan (blood work).

___27. discussed precautions necessary so as not to infect others.

___28. stated that the girlfriend should be examined by a physician.

If you performed 20 of these 28 tasks, you passed this test station.

You have 10 minutes to complete your patient note.

HISTORY—Include significant positives and negatives from the history of present illness, past medical history, review of systems, and social and family history.

_____

_____

_____

_____

_____

_____

_____

_____

_____

PHYSICAL EXAMINATION—Indicate only the pertinent positive and negative findings related to the patient's chief complaint.

_____

_____

_____

_____

_____

_____

_____

_____

_____

_____

DIFFERENTIAL DIAGNOSIS—In order of likelihood, write no more than five differential diagnoses for this patient's current problems.

1. _____

2. _____

3. _____

4. _____

5. _____

DIAGNOSTIC WORKUP—Immediate plans for no more than five diagnostic studies.

1. _____

2. _____

3. _____

4. _____

5. _____

A SATISFACTORY PATIENT NOTE

HISTORY—Include significant positives and negatives from the history of present illness, past medical history, review of systems, and social and family history.

Mr. Donald Dearborn is a 25-year-old college student with a 7-day history of fever and swollen tender neck glands. He has had temperatures as high as 101.5°F and a sore throat but denies coughing. He has no abdominal pain but feels as if his upper abdomen has become swollen and he has lost his appetite. He has no nausea, vomiting, or change in bowel movements. Since yesterday he has noticed that his eyes and skin have turned a yellow color. He has no past medical history of jaundice, hepatitis, blood transfusion, body piercing, tattoos or eating shellfish. He does not drink, smoke cigarettes, or use illicit drugs. He takes no medications and has no recent travel. He is sexually active in a monogamous relationship with his girlfriend who is experiencing similar symptoms. He is heterosexual, has had two previous sexual partners, and always uses condoms. He received hepatitis B vaccination prior to starting college.

PHYSICAL EXAMINATION—Indicate only the pertinent positive and negative findings related to the patient's chief complaint.

Patient is a well-developed young man in no acute distress. He appears, however, concerned and anxious.
Vital signs are significant for a temperature of 101.2°F
Skin: No spider angiomata or palmar erythema. Positive for jaundice.
HEENT: PERLA. EOMI. Sclerae icteric. Conjunctivae pink. throat erythematous without exudate. Tender but freely movable bilateral posterior cervical lymphadenopathy. No supraclavicular lymphadenopathy.
Heart and lungs: Normal.
Abdomen: Normal bowel sounds. Liver 14 cm in midclavicular line by percussion. Diffuse tenderness with palpation over right and left upper quadrants.
Neuro: No deficits.

DIFFERENTIAL DIAGNOSIS

In order of likelihood, write no more than five differential diagnoses for this patient's current problems.

1. mononucleosis
2. hepatitis A
3. hepatitis B
4. hepatitis C
5. Gilbert's syndrome

DIAGNOSTIC WORKUP

Immediate plans for no more than five diagnostic studies.

1. CBC for atypical lymphocytes
2. liver function tests (unconjugated and conjugated bilirubin, AST, ALT, alkaline phosphatase)
3. monospot test
4. hepatitis A, B, and C serology
5. ultrasound of liver

LEARNING OBJECTIVE FOR MR. DEARBORN
RECOGNIZE THE RISK FACTORS AND POSSIBLE ETIOLOGIES
IN A PATIENT WITH NEW-ONSET JAUNDICE

Infectious mononucleosis is an acute disease due to Epstein-Barr virus (herpesvirus) that commonly occurs in individuals who are 10 to 35 years of age. The symptoms of this disease are so variable that it is often difficult to form a narrow and focused differential diagnosis. Fever, anorexia, sore throat, and tender posterior cervical lymphadenopathy are the common symptoms on presentation.

Mr. Dearborn is a young man who presented with the complaints of fever, sore throat, and tender cervical lymphadenopathy. He denied having a cough, so a respiratory infection is less likely to explain his symptoms.

The patient presented with new-onset jaundice but denied having the common risk factors for viral hepatitis, such as a past medical history of blood transfusion, illicit drug use, body piercing, tattoos, and sexual promiscuity. He denied having the risk factors for hepatitis A virus. He has been vaccinated against hepatitis B. He uses no medications that may have caused hepatotoxicity. He denies alcohol abuse; therefore alcoholic hepatitis is unlikely.

The abdominal fullness without associated gastrointestinal symptoms, the jaundice, and the tender liver on physical examination may be seen with many diseases, including infectious mononucleosis. The patient may still have viral hepatitis, and serology will be performed for hepatitis A, B, and C once infectious mononucleosis is ruled out.

The patient's girlfriend's having similar symptomatology is significant, since the mode of transmission of mononucleosis is through saliva. The doctor should recommend that the patient's girlfriend be seen by a physician and evaluated for infectious mononucleosis.

A complete blood profile on Mr. Dearborn would most likely reveal a predominance of atypical lymphocytes, and a monospot test (IgM) would confirm the diagnosis. Even though mononucleosis has a benign course, its possible complications (mononeuritis, encephalitis, cardiac arrhythmia) and infectious precautions must be discussed with each patient.

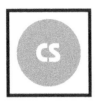

Patient Note Pearl: The **differential diagnosis** for this patient would include mononucleosis, hepatitis A, B, C, and alcoholic hepatitis. Rotor's syndrome and Dubin-Johnson syndrome cause elevation of conjugated bilirubin and may produce jaundice (Gilbert's syndrome produces elevation of unconjugated bilirubin). Jaundice may also be due to disorders of bilirubin metabolism, such as hemolytic anemia and sickle cell disease. Posthepatic causes of jaundice include gallstones, biliary stricture, and primary sclerosing cholangitis. The **diagnostic workup** includes a peripheral blood smear to identify atypical lymphocytes, a monospot test, and bilirubin (unconjugated and conjugated levels), aspartate aminotransferase (AST), alanine aminotransferase (ALT), and alkaline phosphatase levels.

NOTES

Case 6

A 68-year-old man named David Dubois recently moved to the small town where you are the only practicing physician. He was diagnosed with pancreatic cancer 7 months ago and knows he is dying. He wants you to be his physician for the remaining days or months of his life.

As you enter the examination room, you notice a frail and cachectic man looking much older than his 68 years. He is jaundiced. He is requesting a prescription for narcotics.

Vital Signs:

Temperature	98.2°F.
Blood pressure	115/75 mmHg
Heart rate	88 beats per minute
Respiratory rate	14 breaths per minute

Examinee's Tasks

1. Obtain a focused and relevant history.
2. Discuss your plan for pain management with the patient.
3. Discuss death and dying issues with patient.
4. After seeing the patient, complete paperwork relevant to the case.

MY CHECKLIST

History of Present Illness. The Examinee:

1. _____
2. _____
3. _____
4. _____
   _____
5. _____
6. _____
   _____
7. _____
8. _____
9. _____
10. _____
    _____
11. _____
    _____
12. _____
13. _____

Communication Skills. The Examinee:

14. _____
15. _____
16. _____
17. _____
18. _____
19. _____
20. _____
    _____
21. _____
22. _____
23. _____
24. _____
25. _____
26. _____

SP CHECKLIST FOR MR. DUBOIS

History of Present Illness. The Examinee:

___ 1. started with an open-ended question, i.e., "What is troubling you, Mr. Dubois?"

___ 2. asked about appetite, i.e., worsening weight loss ("I just don't have the strength to eat anything.")

___ 3. asked about recent fevers ("None.")

___ 4. asked about any pain ("This cancer causes a lot of pain in my whole body; I definitely need more pain medication.")

___ 5. asked about any other medical problems ("None.")

___ 6. asked about present medications ("I take morphine pills twice a day; they aren't strong enough, though; I need a higher dose; will you give me a stronger prescription?")

___ 7. asked about my support system, i.e., family and friends ("I really have no one; I'm all alone in this world.")

___ 8. asked about home situation ("I live alone.")

___ 9. asked if I needed help at home ("I could use a little help now and then with shopping, cooking, and cleaning.")

___10. asked about a proxy for health decisions or a durable power of attorney for health decisions ("I really have no one but I want nothing done; just make sure I die in peace.")

___11. asked about family history of cancer ("Yes my father and brother died of pancreatic cancer and there is no way I am going to suffer like they did.")

___12. asked about smoking cigarettes ("No, never did.")

___13. asked about alcohol use ("No.")

Communication Skills. The Examinee:

___14. greeted me warmly.

___15. introduced self to me.

___16. created an atmosphere of trust and respect.

___17. made good eye contact.

___18. used appropriate body language.

___19. adapted personal style of speech to my needs.

___20. asked me about advance directives, i.e., living will ("Yes; I want to have one of those; I wish to die at home in peace without pain.")

___21. stated would increase the pain medication ("Oh, thank you, Doctor.")

___22. stated would help me to die at home ("Oh, thank you, Doctor.")

___23. offered hospice involvement ("Oh, thank you, Doctor.")

___24. addressed my concerns.

___25. showed interest in me as a person.

___26. offered ongoing partnership and support.

If you performed 19 of these 26 tasks, you passed this test station.

You have 10 minutes to complete your patient note.

HISTORY—Include significant positives and negatives from the history of present illness, past medical history, review of systems, and social and family history.

_____

_____

_____

_____

_____

_____

_____

_____

_____

_____

PHYSICAL EXAMINATION—Indicate only the pertinent positive and negative findings related to the patient's chief complaint.

_____

_____

_____

_____

_____

_____

_____

_____

_____

_____

DIFFERENTIAL DIAGNOSIS—In order of likelihood, write no more than five differential diagnoses for this patient's current problems.

1. _____

2. _____

3. _____

4. _____

5. _____

DIAGNOSTIC WORKUP—Immediate plans for no more than five diagnostic studies.

1. _____

2. _____

3. _____

4. _____

5. _____

A SATISFACTORY PATIENT NOTE

HISTORY—Include significant positives and negatives from the history of present illness, past medical history, review of systems, and social and family history.

Mr. Dubois is a 68-year-old man with a history of pancreatic cancer that was diagnosed 7 months ago. He is aware of his poor prognosis and wishes the physician to assist him with terminal care and pain management. He has a decreased appetite and has been losing weight. He denies fever. He takes morphine pills twice a day but still has pain and wants stronger pain medications. He has no other medical problems. The patient is living alone, has no real support system, and would be accepting of a home health aide to assist with the shopping, laundering, housekeeping and cooking. He has no durable power of attorney for health care decisions or a health care proxy. The patient is interested in completing a living will or advance directive stating that he wishes to die in the comfort of his own home. He would be accepting of hospice care should he need that kind of support and assistance. Mr. Dubois does not smoke cigarettes or drink alcohol. He has a family history that is positive for his father and only sibling dying of pancreatic cancer.

PHYSICAL EXAMINATION—Indicate only the pertinent positive and negative findings related to the patient's chief complaint.

Vital signs are normal. Patient is frail and cachectic. NAD.

DIFFERENTIAL DIAGNOSIS
In order of likelihood, write no more than five differential diagnoses for this patient's current problems.

1. pancreatic cancer
2. palliative/terminal care
3. pain management
4.
5.

DIAGNOSTIC WORKUP
Immediate plans for no more than five diagnostic studies.

1. advance directive
2. hospice
3. CBC
4. electrolytes
5. pancreatic support group

LEARNING OBJECTIVE FOR MR. DUBOIS
DISCUSSING END-OF-LIFE ISSUES WITH A DYING PATIENT

Mr. Dubois has accepted his diagnosis of pancreatic cancer and wants his doctor to help him with terminal care. His wish is to die at home without pain. He seeks a physician willing to discuss advance directives and hospice care. He wants a physician who will not hesitate to increase his pain medications even if higher doses of narcotics may hasten his death. Pain is Mr. Dubois's greatest fear about dying. During the interview, the physician should inquire about symptoms the patient may be having secondary to the malignancy. Mr. Dubois admits to anorexia and weight loss but denies having fever or other signs of infection. He complains of diffuse body pain.

The physician should ask about preexisting medical problems or comorbid conditions that may require future treatment. Mr. Dubois denies having any past medical history.

The social history should include a discussion about the patient's existing support system. Does the patient have friends and family? What is the home situation like for this patient? Arrange for community resources to assist this dying patient if necessary.

A physician discussing end-of-life decisions must allow the patient an opportunity to state concerns and ask questions. A patient's nonverbal clues should be acknowledged and addressed. There must be an atmosphere of trust and respect between the patient and physician.

The physician must state that he or she will respect the wishes of the patient. The physician should not be concerned about hastening the patient's death with narcotics. The physician must promise to increase pain medications to relieve the patient's suffering and pain. Competent and informed patients must be given the dignity and autonomy to make end-of-life decisions.

History-Taking Pearl: Remember to ask the patient about a durable power of attorney for health care decisions or a health care proxy in addition to the living will.

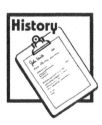

Patient Note Pearl: Sometimes in the CS, the **differential diagnosis** may not go beyond one or two diagnoses. In this case, for example, it is sufficient to write pancreatic cancer, palliative care, and terminal pain as the differential diagnosis. **Diagnostic workup** might include CBC (for anemia) and baseline electrolytes, amylase, and lipase. You may also want to arrange for a living will, health care proxy, and pancreatic cancer support group.

Case 7

You are instructed to see Mrs. Dolores Darling, a 50-year-old security guard. She has not seen a physician in 5 years. Recently, she went to a health fair and, after a free blood pressure check, was told to see a physician for possible high blood pressure. Your name was in her managed care book, so she made an appointment to see you. This is her first visit.

Vital Signs:

Temperature	98.6°F
Blood pressure	150/95 mmHg
Heart rate	80 beats per minute
Respiratory rate	12 breaths per minute

You enter the examination room and see an obese female (210 pounds with a height of 63 inches). She is in no distress.

Examinee's Tasks

1. Obtain a focused and relevant history.
2. Perform a focused and relevant physical examination.
3. Discuss your initial diagnostic impressions with the patient.
4. Discuss follow-up tests with the patient.
5. After seeing the patient, complete paperwork relevant to the case.

MY CHECKLIST

History of Present Illness. The Examinee:

1. _____
   _____
2. _____
3. _____
4. _____
5. _____
6. _____
7. _____
8. _____
9. _____
   _____
10. _____

Physical Examination. The Examinee:

11. _____
12. _____
13. _____
    _____
14. _____
15. _____
16. _____
17. _____
18. _____
19. _____

Communication Skills. The Examinee:

20. _____
21. _____
22. _____
23. _____
24. _____
25. _____
26. _____
    _____
27. _____
28. _____
29. _____

SP CHECKLIST FOR MRS. DARLING

History of Present Illness. The Examinee:

___ 1. asked about any symptoms, i.e., headaches, blurred vision, palpitations, shortness of breath, chest pain, dizziness ("No.")

___ 2. asked about past medical history ("None.")

___ 3. asked about medication use ("None.")

___ 4. asked about diet ("I eat a lot of junk food.")

___ 5. asked about tobacco use ("I've smoked two packs per day for 20 years.")

___ 6. asked about illicit drug use ("Never.")

___ 7. asked about exercise ("None.")

___ 8. asked about stresses in life, i.e., employment or family ("None.")

___ 9. asked about family history ("My father had a heart attack at the age of 60, and my mother suffered a stroke at the age of 65; a sister who is 50 years old has congestive heart failure and diabetes.")

___10. asked if cholesterol level is known ("At the fair, they told me my cholesterol was 300. Is that high?")

Physical Examination. The Examinee:

___11. checked my blood pressure in both arms (blood pressure in both arms is 150/95 mmHg).

___12. checked my blood pressure sitting and standing (blood pressure is 150/95 mmHg).

___13. chose the large cuff to measure my blood pressure (examination room had a small and a large cuff available for the examinee to choose from).

___12. looked into eyes with ophthalmoscope (normal examination).

___13. Felt my thyroid gland (normal)

___14. palpated front of chest to feel for point of maximum impulse (PMI).

___15. listened to heart in at least three places (normal examination).

___16. listened to lungs in at least four places (normal examination).

___17. listened over abdomen with stethoscope (no bruits audible).

___18. palpated sides of abdomen to determine kidney size (kidneys not enlarged).

___19. felt at least two of my pulses, i.e., carotid, radial, posterior tibialis, dorsalis pedis (normal pulses are palpable).

Communication Skills. The Examinee:

___20. created an atmosphere that put me at ease.

___21. explained the results of the physical examination.

___22. discussed all my medical problems (hypertension, hyperlipidemia, obesity, tobacco use).

___23. discussed diet as a treatment for hypertension, obesity, and hyperlipidemia.

___24. discussed exercise as a treatment for hypertension, obesity, and hyperlipidemia.

___25. educated me regarding prognosis if problems are left untreated.

___26. discussed structured plan (blood work, urinalysis, electrocardiogram, exercise program, nutrition guidelines, tobacco cessation program).

___27. inquired about my understanding of the problems.

___28. inquired whether I would comply with the plan.

___29. appeared supportive and confident that I would succeed.

If you performed 21 of these 29 tasks, you passed this test station.

You have 10 minutes to complete your patient note.

HISTORY—Include significant positives and negatives from the history of present illness, past medical history, review of systems, and social and family history.

_____
_____
_____
_____
_____
_____
_____
_____
_____
_____
_____

PHYSICAL EXAMINATION—Indicate only the pertinent positive and negative findings related to the patient's chief complaint.

_____
_____
_____
_____
_____
_____
_____
_____
_____
_____
_____

DIFFERENTIAL DIAGNOSIS—In order of likelihood, write no more than five differential diagnoses for this patient's current problems.

1. _____
2. _____
3. _____
4. _____
5. _____

DIAGNOSTIC WORKUP—Immediate plans for no more than five diagnostic studies.

1. _____
2. _____
3. _____
4. _____
5. _____

A SATISFACTORY PATIENT NOTE

HISTORY—Include significant positives and negatives from the history of present illness, past medical history, review of systems, and social and family history.

The patient is a 50-year old security guard who was advised at a health fair to see a private doctor for possible high blood pressure. The patient denies any headaches, blurred vision, chest pain, palpitations, or shortness of breath. She has no past medical history and takes no medications. She smokes two packs of cigarettes per day but does not drink alcohol or use drugs. Her diet consists of "junk food" and she is sedentary. She describes her life as low stress and has no problems with her family or employment. Family history is positive for diabetes, myocardial infarction, stroke, and congestive heart failure. The patient states that at the health fair, she was informed that her cholesterol level was over 300.

PHYSICAL EXAMINATION—Indicate only the pertinent positive and negative findings related to the patient's chief complaint.

The patient is cooperative and in no acute distress. She is morbidly obese. She is not hirsute and has no acne.
BP right arm = 150/95 mmHg. BP left arm = 150/95 mmHg
BP lying down: right arm = 150/95 mmHg. BP standing: right arm = 150/95 mmHg.
Weight = 210 lb. height = 63 in. BMI = $210/(63)^2 \times 703 = 37.20 \text{ kg/m}^2$.
HEENT: PERLA. EOMI. Fundi = no exudates, hemorrhages, or papilledema. Thyroid normal. No JVD. No carotid bruits.
Heart: PMI 5th ICS MCL. Normal heart sounds. No murmurs or gallops.
Lungs: Clear to auscultation and percussion.
Abdomen: Normal BS. No masses. Kidneys not palpable. No epigastric bruits.
Extremities: No edema. Pulses 2+ bilaterally
Neuro: Alert and oriented × 3. No deficits.

DIFFERENTIAL DIAGNOSIS

In order of likelihood, write no more than five differential diagnoses for this patient's current problems.

1. essential hypertension
2. morbid obesity
3. r/o hypothyroidism
4. hyperlipidemia
5. tobacco addiction

DIAGNOSTIC WORKUP

Immediate plans for no more than five diagnostic studies.

1. CBC
2. electrolytes
3. lipid profile
4. electrocardiogram
5. TSH level

LEARNING OBJECTIVE FOR MRS. DARLING
APPROACH TO THE PATIENT WHO PRESENTS WITH HYPERTENSION

Even though patients with hypertension are usually asymptomatic, when a patient presents with hypertension, the physician should inquire about headaches, dizziness, blurred vision, palpitations, chest pain, and shortness of breath. If a secondary cause of hypertension is suspected, such as Cushing's disease (hirsutism, facial plethora, truncal obesity, headache, acne) or pheochromocytoma (headache, palpitations, diaphoresis), the physician should inquire about the symptoms specific to those diseases.

Risk factors that contribute to hypertension include a past medical history of hyperlipidemia or diabetes mellitus and the use of medications such as estrogen in oral contraceptives. A patient must be asked about a family history of cardiac disease or hyperlipidemia. The physician should inquire about tobacco and cocaine use. A patient's lifestyle can affect blood pressure and the physician should inquire about diet, exercise, living arrangements, and stressful employment.

Blood pressure readings should be measured twice during two separate examinations with the appropriate size cuff before making the diagnosis of hypertension. Both arms should be used to record blood pressure (pressure in one arm may be lower due to a narrow brachial/axillary artery and, in the future, the arm with the higher recording should be used). Blood pressure should be measured sitting and standing to identify patients with orthostatic hypotension.

A funduscopic examination may reveal information about the duration of the hypertension. The heart examination may reveal a murmur, gallop, or displaced point of maximum impulse (PMI). A lung examination may reveal cardiac decompensation. The abdominal examination is required for palpation of enlarged kidneys secondary to polycystic renal disease and to auscultate for renal artery bruits. Peripheral pulses should be palpated for diminished flow secondary to atherosclerosis.

Risk-factor modification and patient compliance must be addressed in treating a patient with hypertension. Mrs. Darling should be encouraged to stop smoking, increase her physical activity, and reduce her salt and fat intake in an effort to lose weight. She should be educated about the complications of untreated hypertension and the importance of compliance and follow-up.

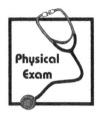

Physical Examination Pearl: Know that patients <25 or >45 years old with new hypertension should be examined closely for secondary causes of hypertension (pheochromocytoma, renal artery stenosis, hyperaldosteronism, Cushing's disease, polycystic kidney disease, coarctation of the aorta, hyperparathyroidism, thyroid disease, acromegaly), even though these are responsible for less than 5 percent of all hypertension.

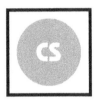

Patient Note Pearl: The **workup** for hypertension includes a hematocrit, serum glucose level, potassium level, creatinine level, urinalysis for protein and blood, and an electrocardiogram. Special studies to screen for secondary causes of hypertension should be ordered when necessary.

NOTES

Case 8

Please evaluate Mr. Michael Brown, a 55-year-old construction worker, with the chief complaint of abdominal pain. He has a 10-year history of hypertension well controlled with an angiotensin-converting enzyme (ACE) inhibitor. The physician assistant reports that the rectal examination revealed no masses but was positive for occult blood.

Vital Signs:

Temperature	98.6°F
Blood pressure	120/80 mmHg
Heart rate	80 beats per minute
Respiratory rate	12 breaths per minute

Examinee's Tasks

1. Obtain a focused and relevant history.
2. Perform a focused and relevant physical examination.
3. Discuss your initial diagnostic impressions with the patient.
4. Discuss follow-up tests with the patient.
5. After seeing the patient, complete paperwork relevant to the case.

MY CHECKLIST

History of Present Illness. The Examinee:

1. _____
2. _____
3. _____
4. _____
5. _____
6. _____
7. _____
8. _____
9. _____
10. _____
11. _____
12. _____
13. _____
14. _____
15. _____

Physical Examination. The Examinee:

16. _____
17. _____
18. _____
19. _____

Communication Skills. The Examinee:

20. _____
21. _____
22. _____
23. _____
24. _____
    _____
25. _____

SP CHECKLIST FOR MR. BROWN

History of Present Illness. The Examinee:

___ 1. asked about onset of pain ("It has been about 2 months.")
___ 2. asked about location of pain ("In the upper part of my abdomen.")
___ 3. asked about the quality of the pain ("Burning and gnawing in nature.")
___ 4. asked about radiation of pain ("None.")
___ 5. asked if the pain was constant or intermittent ("Mostly it's there all the time.")
___ 6. asked about the severity of the pain ("On a scale of 1 to 10, where 10 is the worst, the pain is a 3.")
___ 7. asked about any aggravating factors ("Alcohol, caffeine, smoking, stress, and not eating make it worse.")
___ 8. asked about any alleviating factors ("Food and antacids make it better.")
___ 9. asked about any association with nausea or vomiting ("None.")
___10. asked about any change in bowel movements ("No diarrhea or constipation.")
___11. asked about blood in the stools or tarry stools ("No.")
___12. asked about alcohol use ("Just a beer on Sundays.")
___13. asked about tobacco use ("I smoke a pack per day.")
___14. asked about frequent aspirin or nonsteroidal pain medication use ("No.")
___15. asked about weight loss ("None.")

Physical Examination. The Examinee:

___16. performed orthostatics (blood pressure and heart rate do not change from laying to standing position)
___17. listened over the abdomen with a stethoscope (normal bowel sounds are heard).
___18. pressed gently on abdomen (SP will complain of mild pain in epigastric area).
___19. pressed deeply on abdomen (SP will complain of marked pain in epigastric area).

Communication Skills. The Examinee:

___20. explained the results of the physical examination.
___21. discussed the plausible diagnosis (ulcer or gastritis).
___22. discussed the follow-up steps in management (blood work, gastroenterology consultation for endoscopy).
___23. discussed treatment options (will need medications and follow-up).
___24. recommended abstinence from alcohol, tobacco, aspirin, nonsteroidal anti-inflammatory drugs, and caffeine-containing beverages.
___25. discussed prognosis with me (good prognosis).

If you performed 18 of these 25 tasks, you passed this test station.

You have 10 minutes to complete your patient note.

HISTORY—Include significant positives and negatives from the history of present illness, past medical history, review of systems, and social and family history.

_____

_____

_____

_____

_____

_____

_____

_____

_____

_____

_____

PHYSICAL EXAMINATION—Indicate only the pertinent positive and negative findings related to the patient's chief complaint.

_____

_____

_____

_____

_____

_____

_____

_____

_____

_____

_____

DIFFERENTIAL DIAGNOSIS—In order of likelihood, write no more than five differential diagnoses for this patient's current problems.

1. _____

2. _____

3. _____

4. _____

5. _____

DIAGNOSTIC WORKUP—Immediate plans for no more than five diagnostic studies.

1. _____

2. _____

3. _____

4. _____

5. _____

A SATISFACTORY PATIENT NOTE

HISTORY—Include significant positives and negatives from the history of present illness, past medical history, review of systems, and social and family history.

Mr. Michael Brown is a 55-year-old construction worker who presents with the chief complaint of abdominal pain for 2 months. The pain is located in the epigastric area and is burning and gnawing in nature. The pain does not radiate. On a scale of 1 to 10, he describes the pain as being a 3. The pain is constant but is aggravated by alcohol, caffeine, smoking, stress, and not eating. The pain is alleviated by food and antacids. He denies nausea, vomiting, diarrhea, constipation, and weight loss. He denies melena and hematochezia. The patient smokes a pack of cigarettes per day and drinks one beer every Sunday. He does not take aspirin or NSAIDs. Past medical history is significant for hypertension which is well-controlled with an ACE inhibitor.

PHYSICAL EXAMINATION—Indicate only the pertinent positive and negative findings related to the patient's chief complaint.

Well-developed and well-nourished man who looks his stated age of 55 afebrile in no acute distress
BP = 120/80 mm Hg laying down. BP = 123/82 mmHg standing
HR = 84 beats/min laying down. HR = 85 beats/min standing
HEENT: PERLA. Conjunctiva pink. Sclerae nonicteric
Lungs: Clear to auscultation and percussion
Heart: Normal heart sounds. No murmurs or gallops
Abdomen: Normal BS. Liver size in MCL 12 cm. No splenomegaly. Nontender. No rebound, rigidity or guarding.
Rectal: Fecal occult blood positive. No masses.

DIFFERENTIAL DIAGNOSIS
In order of likelihood, write no more than five differential diagnoses for this patient's current problems.

1. peptic ulcer disease
2. nonulcer dyspepsia
3. gastritis
4. pancreatitis
5. malignancy

DIAGNOSTIC WORKUP
Immediate plans for no more than five diagnostic studies.

1. CBC
2. amylase and lipase
3. upper barium gastrointestinal study
4. *H. pylori* urease breath test
5. endoscopy (EGD)

LEARNING OBJECTIVE FOR MR. BROWN
EVALUATE CHRONIC ABDOMINAL PAIN IN PATIENT
WITH HEME POSITIVE STOOLS

This patient presents with a 2-month history of epigastric discomfort relieved with food and antacids. He appears to be in no acute distress and is afebrile. His mild and infrequent abdominal pain is alleviated with antacids and food and is aggravated by stress, caffeine, tobacco, and mild alcohol use.

Mr. Brown denies a history of weight loss or a change in bowel movements, but malignancy must remain a consideration in someone with heme-positive stools. Pancreatitis is unlikely, since the epigastric pain does not radiate to the back, is relieved with food, and is not associated with nausea or vomiting. Peptic ulcer disease and gastritis remain plausible considerations and require further investigation in this patient.

There are 500,000 new cases of peptic ulcer disease in the United States each year. The disease occurs more commonly in men than in women. *Helicobacter pylori* and the use of NSAIDs are the main etiologies of ulcer disease. The most common complaint in a patient with ulcer is epigastric discomfort or dyspepsia. Fecal blood testing in patients with peptic ulcer is positive in 30 percent.

The physician should evaluate Mr. Brown for chronic blood loss by ordering a hematocrit. A gastroenterology consultation for endoscopy with antral biopsy to determine whether *H. pylori* is present would be the most accurate method to diagnose ulcer and exclude malignancy. If ulcer disease and *H. pylori* infection are confirmed, the patient will need antibiotics combined with acid suppression therapy. The patient should attempt to abstain from using tobacco, alcohol, and caffeine-containing beverages.

Patient Note Pearl: The **differential diagnosis** for a patient with chronic abdominal pain includes peptic ulcer disease, nonulcer dyspepsia, gastritis, pancreatitis, and malignancy. The **diagnostic workup** includes a fecal occult blood test, CBC, and possibly amylase and lipase. Other tests to consider include a gastroenterology consult for endoscopy with antral biopsy, upper barium gastrointestinal study (80 percent accurate for gastric and duodenal ulcers) and *H. pylori* by the urease breath test (95 percent sensitive) or serum antibodies (95 percent sensitive but not able to distinguish between past and present infection).

Case 9

Mr. Louis Levitt, 48 years old, is complaining of chest pain.

Vital Signs:

Temperature	98.6°F
Blood pressure	140/90 mmHg
Heart rate	100 beats per minute
Respiratory rate	16 breaths per minute

Examinee's Tasks

1. Obtain a focused and relevant history.
2. Perform a focused and relevant physical examination.
3. Discuss your initial diagnostic impressions with the patient.
4. Discuss follow-up tests with the patient.
5. After seeing the patient, complete paperwork relevant to the case.

MY CHECKLIST

History of Present Illness. The Examinee:

1. _____
2. _____
3. _____
4. _____
5. _____
6. _____
7. _____
8. _____
9. _____
10. _____
11. _____
12. _____
13. _____
14. _____
15. _____
16. _____
17. _____

Physical Examination. The Examinee:

18. _____
19. _____
20. _____
21. _____

Communication Skills. The Examinee:

22. _____
23. _____
24. _____
25. _____
26. _____
27. _____
28. _____

SP CHECKLIST FOR MR. LEVITT

History of Present Illness. The Examinee:

___ 1. asked about the location of the chest pain ("In the middle of my chest.")

___ 2. asked about the quality of the chest pain ("It almost feels like indigestion.")

___ 3. asked about the onset of the chest pain ("Started about 1 hour ago while I was working at my desk.")

___ 4. asked about the severity of the chest pain ("On a scale of 1 to 10 where 10 is the worst, this is a 7.")

___ 5. asked about radiation of the pain ("It goes to my left arm.")

___ 6. asked what makes the chest pain worse ("Walking makes it worse.")

___ 7. asked what makes the chest pain better ("Nothing really.")

___ 8. asked if pain was associated with nausea or vomiting ("I do feel nauseated right now.")

___ 9. asked about other symptoms, i.e., shortness of breath, palpitations, and dizziness ("No, none of that.")

___10. asked about past medical history ("Never ill before; have not seen a doctor in 10 years.")

___11. asked about tobacco use ("I've smoked two packs per day for 15 years.")

___12. asked about cocaine use ("No.")

___13. asked about alcohol use ("Rarely.")

___14. asked about diet ("I eat junk food.")

___15. asks about exercise ("No, I have no time to exercise.")

___16. asked about family history ("My brother and father died of heart attacks before the age of 60.")

___17. asked about lifestyle stresses, i.e., family or occupation ("I work as a stockbroker on Wall Street; it is a stressful job.")

Physical Examination. The Examinee:

___18. palpated my precordium for the PMI (normal).

___19. listened to my heart in at least three places (normal heart exam).

___20. listened to my lungs in at least four places (lung examination is normal).

___21. evaluated my neck veins looking for elevation of pressure (no jugular venous distention).

Communication Skills. The Examinee:

___22. made me feel at ease.

___23. conveyed confidence.

___24. alleviated my fears.

___25. explained the diagnostic possibilities to me (i.e., myocardial infarction, unstable angina, pericarditis).

___26. explained the workup [electrocardiogram, chest x-ray (CXR), bloodwork].

___27. gave me sublingual nitroglycerin and aspirin.

___28. discussed the risk factors that contribute to a cardiac problem (smoking, family history, diet, sedentary lifestyle, and stress).

If you performed 20 of these 28 tasks, you passed this test station.

You have 10 minutes to complete your patient note.

HISTORY—Include significant positives and negatives from the history of present illness, past medical history, review of systems, and social and family history.

_____
_____
_____
_____
_____
_____
_____
_____
_____
_____
_____

PHYSICAL EXAMINATION—Indicate only the pertinent positive and negative findings related to the patient's chief complaint.

_____
_____
_____
_____
_____
_____
_____
_____
_____
_____
_____

DIFFERENTIAL DIAGNOSIS—In order of likelihood, write no more than five differential diagnoses for this patient's current problems.

1. _____
2. _____
3. _____
4. _____
5. _____

DIAGNOSTIC WORKUP—Immediate plans for no more than five diagnostic studies.

1. _____
2. _____
3. _____
4. _____
5. _____

A SATISFACTORY PATIENT NOTE

HISTORY—Include significant positives and negatives from the history of present illness, past medical history, review of systems, and social and family history.

Mr. Louis Levitt is a 48-year-old wall street stockbroker who presents to the emergency room with a one-hour history of substernal chest pain which he describes as being similar to indigestion. He states that the chest pain is a 7 on a scale of 1 to 10. The pain radiates to his left arm and is associated with nausea. Nothing seems to alleviate the pain, but it was aggravated by walking around the office prior to coming to the emergency room. He denies shortness of breath, dizziness, vomiting, and palpitations. The patient has no past medical history and has not seen a physician in 10 years. He smokes two packs of cigarettes a day for over 15 years but does not use cocaine or drink alcohol. His diet consists of mostly junk food and his lifestyle is sedentary. Family history is significant for a brother and father dying of heart attacks in their fifties.

PHYSICAL EXAMINATION—Indicate only the pertinent positive and negative findings related to the patient's chief complaint.

The patient is overweight (approximately 5'9" tall and 210 pounds) and looks older than his stated age of 48 years. He is extremely anxious and uncomfortable lying on the stretcher. He is very diaphoretic.
BP = 140/90 mmHg right arm. BP = 145/92 mmHg left arm.
HR = 100 beats/min and regular. RR = 16.
HEENT: PERLA. No JVD. Thyroid normal.
Lungs: Clear to auscultation.
Heart: PMI 5th ICS MCL. Normal S_1 and S_2. No gallops, rubs, or murmurs.
Abdomen: Normal bowel sounds. Nontender.
Extremities: No cyanosis or edema. Peripheral pulses 2+ diffusely.

DIFFERENTIAL DIAGNOSIS
In order of likelihood, write no more than five differential diagnoses for this patient's current problems.

1. myocardial infarction
2. angina
3. aortic dissection
4. pulmonary embolus
5. pericarditis

DIAGNOSTIC WORKUP
Immediate plans for no more than five diagnostic studies.

1. electrocardiogram
2. troponin and CPK-MB levels
3. CXR
4. lipid profile
5. echocardiogram

LEARNING OBJECTIVE FOR MR. LEVITT
ASSESSMENT OF THE PATIENT PRESENTING WITH CHEST PAIN

Mr. Levitt presents with typical symptoms of myocardial infarction. The chest pain he is experiencing feels like indigestion; it radiates to his left arm and is associated with nausea. His risk factors for coronary artery disease include age, tobacco use, family history, lack of exercise, and improper diet. The stress of his occupation may also contribute to his illness.

Other risk factors for myocardial infarction may include obesity, cocaine use, and a past medical history of diabetes mellitus, hypertension, or hyperlipidemia. Mr. Levitt does not have these risk factors.

There are 1.5 million myocardial infarctions in the United States per year. The mortality rate in patients presenting acutely is 30 percent. Patients over the age of 65 years have reduced survival and may present with atypical complaints such as shortness of breath instead of chest pain.

The differential diagnosis of chest pain includes gastrointestinal problems, pericarditis, pulmonary embolus, aortic dissection, and costochondritis. Symptomatology and physical examination often help to distinguish among these etiologies. A cardiac examination in a patient with myocardial infarction may reveal an S_4 gallop. Complicated cases may reveal an S_3 gallop or a systolic murmur consistent with mitral valve dysfunction. Lung congestion is found in cases of myocardial infarction complicated by cardiac decompensation. Laboratory tests for a diagnosis of myocardial infarction include an electrocardiogram and serum cardiac markers. Management strategies include reperfusion therapy using thrombolytic agents or primary angioplasty. Pharmacotherapy for acute infarction includes the use of aspirin, beta blockers, ACE inhibitors, nitrates, antiplatelet agents, and oxygen.

The complications of myocardial infarction include cardiac arrhythmias, persistent ischemia, ventricular dysfunction, ventricular rupture, pericarditis, ventricular septal defect, papillary muscle dysfunction, and post–myocardial infarction syndrome. Patients with persistent complications after infarction are at increased risk of reinfarction and death.

Secondary prevention of myocardial infarction requires the patient to modify all risk factors for atherosclerosis. Mr. Levitt must stop smoking and begin eating a low-fat diet. He must begin an exercise program. The occupational stress of being a Wall Street stockbroker should be reduced if possible.

Patient Note Pearl: The **differential diagnosis** for chest pain includes myocardial infarction, angina, pericarditis, pulmonary embolus, costochondritis, and aortic dissection. Other etiologies may include gastroesophageal reflux disease (GERD), esophageal spasm, cholecystitis, peptic ulcer disease, and herpes zoster. The **diagnostic workup** includes CBC, FOBT, electrocardiography, cardiac isoenzymes including troponin level, CXR, and echocardiogram.

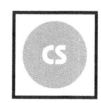

Case 10

You are about to evaluate 25-year-old Ms. Julia Gordon for leg pain.

Vital Signs:

Temperature	98.6°F
Blood pressure	110/70 mmHg
Heart rate	80 beats per minute
Respiratory rate	12 breaths per minute

As you enter the examination room, you notice a thin woman lying on the examination table looking at her right lower extremity.

Examinee's Tasks

1. Obtain a focused and relevant history.
2. Perform a focused and relevant physical examination.
3. Discuss your initial diagnostic impressions with the patient.
4. Discuss follow-up tests with the patient.
5. After seeing the patient, complete paperwork relevant to the case.

MY CHECKLIST

History of Present Illness. The Examinee:

1. _____
2. _____
3. _____
4. _____
5. _____
6. _____
7. _____
8. _____
9. _____
10. _____
11. _____
12. _____
    _____
13. _____

Physical Examination. The Examinee:

14. _____
15. _____
    _____
16. _____
17. _____

Communication Skills. The Examinee:

18. _____
19. _____
20. _____
21. _____
22. _____
23. _____
24. _____

SP CHECKLIST FOR MS. GORDON

History of Present Illness. The Examinee:

___ 1. asked about onset of leg pain ("It started 2 days ago.")
___ 2. asked about trauma to the leg ("No.")
___ 3. asked about any fever ("None.")
___ 4. asked about chest pain ("No.")
___ 5. asked about shortness of breath ("No.")
___ 6. asked if I could be pregnant ("Absolutely not.")
___ 7. asked about past medical history ("Never ill before. I was feeling great until this happened.")
___ 8. asked about medications ("Birth control pills for 7 years.")
___ 9. asked about tobacco use ("I have smoked two packs per day for 5 years.")
___10. asked about illicit drug use ("None.")
___11. asked about family history of blood clots ("No.")
___12. asked about any recent periods of immobilization, i.e., airplane trips ("No, in fact I walk vigorously three times a week; I sometimes walk 5 miles for exercise.")
___13. asked about occupation ("I'm a graduate student majoring in American history.")

Physical Examination. The Examinee:

___14. listened to lungs in at least four places (normal breath sounds are heard).
___15. checked leg for tenderness (right leg will be erythematous and warm to simulate either a deep venous thrombosis (DVT) or a cellulitis; if leg is touched by examinee, SP complains of severe pain).
___16. checked pulse of right foot to confirm good arterial circulation (normal pulse).
___17. checked for a Homans' sign (positive calf pain with passive dorsiflexion of right foot).

Communication Skills. The Examinee:

___18. acknowledged my discomfort.
___19. discussed the diagnostic possibilities in terms I could understand (i.e., DVT, cellulitis, popliteal cyst).
___20. discussed risk factors of tobacco and oral contraceptives for DVT.
___21. checked my understanding of the problem.
___22. discussed plan (bloodwork, venous ultrasonography of leg, admission to the hospital).
___23. discussed treatment with me (anticoagulation with heparin or antibiotics).
___24. discussed prognosis (excellent).

If you performed 17 of these 24 tasks, you passed this test station.

You have 10 minutes to complete your patient note.

HISTORY—Include significant positives and negatives from the history of present illness, past medical history, review of systems, and social and family history.

_____

_____

_____

_____

_____

_____

_____

_____

_____

_____

PHYSICAL EXAMINATION—Indicate only the pertinent positive and negative findings related to the patient's chief complaint.

_____

_____

_____

_____

_____

_____

_____

_____

_____

_____

DIFFERENTIAL DIAGNOSIS—In order of likelihood, write no more than five differential diagnoses for this patient's current problems.

1. _____

2. _____

3. _____

4. _____

5. _____

DIAGNOSTIC WORKUP—Immediate plans for no more than five diagnostic studies.

1. _____

2. _____

3. _____

4. _____

5. _____

A SATISFACTORY PATIENT NOTE

HISTORY—Include significant positives and negatives from the history of present illness, past medical history, review of systems, and social and family history.

Ms. Julia Gordon is a 25-year-old woman with a 2-day history of right leg pain. She denies any trauma to the leg. She has no fever but has noticed that her leg is swollen, warm, and red. She has difficulty ambulating due to the leg pain. She has no past medical history of a similar problem and has never been ill before. She has no recent history of prolonged immobility, such as an airplane or car ride. She is a graduate student majoring in American history and exercises three times a week by walking vigorously. She denies chest pain and shortness of breath. She is not pregnant and has used oral contraceptives for seven years. She takes no other medications. She has smoked 2 ppd for 5 years but does not use illicit drugs. She has no family history of blood clotting problems.

PHYSICAL EXAMINATION—Indicate only the pertinent positive and negative findings related to the patient's chief complaint.

Patient is well developed and well nourished and appears concerned but in NAD. BP = 110/70 mmHg. HR = 80 beats/min. RR = 12 breaths/min. Afebrile.
HT = 66 in. WT = 125 lb. BMI = 20.17 kg/m^2.
Skin: No rashes, ecchymosis, or petechiae.
Lungs: Clear to auscultation and percussion.
Heart: Normal S_1 and S_2. No gallops, rubs or murmurs.
Abdomen: Normal BS. Nontender.
Extremities: RLE erythematous, warm, and tender to palpation. +Homans' sign. Pulses 2+ bilaterally.

DIFFERENTIAL DIAGNOSIS
In order of likelihood, write no more than five differential diagnoses for this patient's current problems.

1. deep venous thrombosis
2. cellulitis
3. popliteal cyst
4. muscle rupture
5.

DIAGNOSTIC WORKUP
Immediate plans for no more than five diagnostic studies.

1. venous ultrasonography of the RLE
2. CBC with platelet count
3. PT, PTT, and INR
4.
5.

LEARNING OBJECTIVE FOR MS. GORDON
APPROACH TO THE PATIENT WITH LEG PAIN

Ms. Gordon presents with an erythematous, warm, and tender right lower extremity, which suggests DVT. She has no complaints or symptoms that suggest a pulmonary embolus.

Her risk factors for DVT include smoking and oral contraceptive use. Other risk factors—including a previous history of DVT, trauma, recent surgery, or a history suggesting malignancy—were denied by the patient. There is no family history of hypercoagulability problems to suggest protein-C resistance (factor V Leiden abnormality), homocystinuria, antiphospholipid antibody syndrome, or deficiencies in protein C, protein S, or antithrombin III. The patient is not obese, and she denies being pregnant. There is no history of prolonged immobilization (airplane trip).

When a patient presents with DVT, the responsible risk factors should be modified when possible to prevent recurrence of clot formation. Ms. Gordon should practice another method of contraception and stop smoking. Every patient with DVT who complains of chest pain or shortness of breath or who presents with tachypnea, tachycardia, or hypoxemia should be urgently investigated for pulmonary embolus. Treatment with anticoagulants is required to prevent the complication of pulmonary embolus.

Patient Note Pearl: The **differential diagnosis** for this patient includes DVT, cellulitis, muscle rupture, lymphedema, ruptured popliteal cyst, and arterial insufficiency. The **diagnostic workup** would include duplex venous ultrasonography to image the deep veins of the leg, CBC with platelet count, prothrombin time (PT), partial thromboplastin time (PTT), and International Normalized Ratio (INR).

Case 11

Mr. Thomas Green is a 35-year-old paramedic. His wife has been your patient for 15 years. She has forced her husband to make an appointment to see you because of his nagging cough.

Vital Signs:

Temperature	100.5°F
Blood pressure	110/70 mmHg
Heart rate	96 beats per minute
Respiratory rate	18 breaths per minute

Upon entering the examination room, you see a thin man in mild respiratory distress coughing continuously.

Examinee's Tasks

1. Obtain a focused and relevant history.
2. Perform a focused and relevant physical examination.
3. Discuss your initial diagnostic impressions with the patient.
4. Discuss follow-up tests with the patient.
5. After seeing the patient, complete paperwork relevant to the case.

MY CHECKLIST

History of Present Illness. The Examinee:

1. _____
2. _____
3. _____
4. _____
5. _____
6. _____
7. _____
8. _____
9. _____
10. _____
11. _____
12. _____
13. _____
_____

Physical Examination. The Examinee:

14. _____
15. _____
16. _____
17. _____
18. _____

Communication Skills. The Examinee:

19. _____
20. _____
21. _____
22. _____
23. _____
24. _____
25. _____

SP CHECKLIST FOR MR. GREEN

History of Present Illness. The Examinee:

___ 1. asked about the onset of cough ("It started about 3 months ago.")

___ 2. asked if cough was productive of sputum ("Yes, some brownish sputum.")

___ 3. asked about blood in the sputum ("Well, I noticed a teaspoon amount of blood yesterday.")

___ 4. asked about any fever ("Lately, my temperature has been 101°F almost every day.")

___ 5. asked about night sweats ("Yes; I have to change my pajamas because I sweat so much at night.")

___ 6. asked about weight loss ("Yes. I've lost 20 pounds in 2 months.")

___ 7. asked about a history of lung problems ("None; no history of asthma, tuberculosis, or pneumonia.")

___ 8. asked about tobacco use ("None.")

___ 9. asked about alcohol use ("No.")

___10. asked about illicit drug use ("No way; are you joking?")

___11. asked about other risk factors for HIV, i.e., promiscuity ("I'm heterosexual and monogamous for 10 years.")

___12. asked about last PPD placement ("8 months ago, and it was negative.") *AKA Mantoux Testing.*

___13. asked about tuberculosis exposure ("I know there are many patients I transport in the ambulance with tuberculosis.")

Physical Examination. The Examinee:

___14. checked my neck for swollen lymph glands (none are palpable).

___15. checked my armpits and above my clavicles for swollen lymph glands (none).

___16. tapped on my back (normal results on percussion of lungs).

___17. listened to my lungs in the front (normal lung sounds are audible).

___18. listened to my lungs in the back (normal lung sounds are audible).

Communication Skills. The Examinee:

___19. shook my hand and introduced self to me.

___20. explained the working diagnosis (tuberculosis or pneumonia; malignancy less likely).

___21. explained the plan (blood work looking for infection, chest radiograph, sputum collection).

___22. asked me to put on a mask as a precaution and explained reason for this to me in a calm manner.

___23. explained that a new PPD would need to be placed now.

___24. explained that, if tuberculosis was diagnosed, close contacts would need to have PPD placement.

___25. offered ongoing support.

If you performed 18 of these 25 tasks, you passed this test station.

You have 10 minutes to complete your patient note.

HISTORY—Include significant positives and negatives from the history of present illness, past medical history, review of systems, and social and family history.

_____
_____
_____
_____
_____
_____
_____
_____
_____
_____
_____

PHYSICAL EXAMINATION—Indicate only the pertinent positive and negative findings related to the patient's chief complaint.

_____
_____
_____
_____
_____
_____
_____
_____
_____
_____
_____

DIFFERENTIAL DIAGNOSIS—In order of likelihood, write no more than five differential diagnoses for this patient's current problems.

1. _____
2. _____
3. _____
4. _____
5. _____

DIAGNOSTIC WORKUP—Immediate plans for no more than five diagnostic studies.

1. _____
2. _____
3. _____
4. _____
5. _____

A SATISFACTORY PATIENT NOTE

HISTORY—Include significant positives and negatives from the history of present illness, past medical history, review of systems, and social and family history.

Mr. Thomas Green is a 35-year-old paramedic with a nagging cough productive of brownish sputum for nearly 3 months. Yesterday he noticed a teaspoon of blood in the sputum. He has been experiencing fevers to 101°F every day and has night sweats that require him to change his pajamas. He has no past medical history of lung problems, such as asthma, tuberculosis, or pneumonia. He has lost approximately 20 pounds in the past 2 months due to a loss of appetite. He does not smoke cigarettes, drink alcohol, or use illicit drugs. He takes no medications. He is heterosexual and monogamous with his wife of 10 years. He is often exposed to patients who have tuberculosis and other illnesses. His PPD, however, was negative 8 months ago.

PHYSICAL EXAMINATION—Indicate only the pertinent positive and negative findings related to the patient's chief complaint.

T = 100.5°F. BP = 110/70 mmHg. HR = 96 beats/min. RR = 18 breaths/min in mild distress. WT = 140 lb. HT = 72 in. BMI = 18.99 kg/m^2. Patient is coughing.
HEENT: No cervical, occipital, submental, or submandibular lymphadenopathy. No axillary or supraclavicular lymphadenopathy.
Lungs: Clear to auscultation and percussion.
Heart: Normal heart sounds.

DIFFERENTIAL DIAGNOSIS
In order of likelihood, write no more than five differential diagnoses for this patient's current problems.

1. tuberculosis
2. pneumonia
3. malignancy
4. asthma
5. COPD

DIAGNOSTIC WORKUP
Immediate plans for no more than five diagnostic studies.

1. CXR
2. PPD placement
3. sputum smear for acid-fast bacilli
4. pulmonary function tests
5.

LEARNING OBJECTIVE FOR MR. GREEN
APPROACH TO THE PATIENT WITH CHRONIC COUGH

Worldwide, there are nearly 4 million new cases of tuberculosis each year. HIV infection, drug use, alcoholism, and poverty have contributed to this large number. Even though his tuberculin skin test was negative in the past, Mr. Green's occupation places him at risk for continuous exposure to tuberculosis.

Although a patient with tuberculosis may be asymptomatic, Mr. Green has symptoms often seen with tuberculosis. He complains of chronic cough with production of brown and bloody sputum, fever, weight loss, and night sweats.

The physical examination of a patient with tuberculosis may be unremarkable. Lymphadenopathy may be absent, and auscultation of the lungs may be normal. The chest radiograph may show apical involvement, but in reality any radiographic abnormality can be seen with tuberculosis.

Mr. Green will need a PPD placement and a chest radiograph. Sputum samples will be collected for smears and culture of acid-fast bacilli. The patient needs to wear a mask (or at least cover his mouth when coughing) to prevent transmission pending the result of the smears. He does not, however, require hospitalization. If tuberculosis is diagnosed, Mr. Green's wife and other close contacts will need a PPD placement and a physician evaluation. This compliant patient can remain at home and be managed as an outpatient.

Patient Note Pearl: The **differential diagnosis** for persistent cough includes tuberculosis, pneumonia, malignancy, asthma, postnasal drip, GERD, chronic obstructive lung disease, bronchiectasis, and certain medications. The **diagnostic workup** may include CXR, PPD placement, sputum for acid-fast bacilli, and pulmonary function tests.

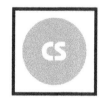

Case 12

A 73-year old woman, Mrs. Eva Divine, presents to the emergency room with the chief complaint of difficulty moving her left arm and leg for the preceding 4 hours.

Vital Signs:

Temperature	98.6°F
Blood pressure	170/110 mmHg
Heart rate	86 beats per minute
Respiratory rate	14 breaths per minute

When you enter the examination room, you see an anxious, tearful patient lying on the examination table.

Examinee's Tasks

1. Obtain a focused and relevant history.
2. Perform a focused and relevant physical examination.
3. Discuss your initial diagnostic impressions with the patient.
4. Discuss follow-up tests with the patient.
5. After seeing the patient, complete paperwork relevant to the case.

MY CHECKLIST

History of Present Illness. The Examinee:

1. _____
2. _____
3. _____
4. _____
5. _____
6. _____
_____
7. _____
8. _____
9. _____
10. _____
11. _____

Physical Examination. The Examinee:

12. _____
13. _____
14. _____
15. _____
_____
16. _____
17. _____
18. _____
19. _____
20. _____
21. _____
22. _____
23. _____
24. _____
25. _____
26. _____

Communication Skills. The Examinee:

27. _____
28. _____
29. _____
30. _____
_____
31. _____
32. _____

SP CHECKLIST FOR MRS. DIVINE

History of Present Illness. The Examinee:

___ 1.   asked about the onset of arm and leg weakness ("It started about 4 hours ago while I was watching television.")

___ 2.   asked about sensory changes in arm and leg ("Yes; the entire arm and leg feel numb.")

___ 3.   asked if my speech was affected ("No but I looked in the mirror and my face looks twisted.")

___ 4.   asked about any cardiac symptoms, i.e., palpitations, irregular heartbeat, chest pain, dizziness, syncope ("No.")

___ 5.   asked about headache or visual changes ("None.")

___ 6.   asked about my past medical history ("I was told by my old doctor that I had borderline high blood pressure but that diet and exercise would help. He told me that I did not need medications.")

___ 7.   asked about a history of diabetes mellitus ("No.")

___ 8.   asked about a history of frequent falls ("No.")

___ 9.   asked about tobacco abuse ("No.")

___10.   asked about alcohol use ("No.")

___11.   asked about occupation ("Retired accountant.")

Physical Examination. The Examinee:

___12.   rechecked blood pressure (170/110 mmHg both arms).

___13.   looked in my eyes with an ophthalmoscope (normal examination).

___14.   checked for visual field cuts with finger wiggling (normal).

___15.   tested the strength in my face, i.e., stick out tongue, grin, squeeze eyes shut (SP will be weak on left side of face when smiling).

___16.   asked me to stick out my tongue (SP will deviate tongue to the left side).

___17.   listened over my neck for carotid bruits (none heard).

___18.   tested the strength in my arms (SP will have a weak left arm).

___19.   tested the strength in my legs (SP will have a weak left leg).

___20.   tested sensation in my arms, i.e., sharp or dull (SP will have decreased sensation in left arm).

___21.   tested sensation in my legs, i.e., sharp or dull (SP will have decreased sensation in left leg).

___22.   tested reflexes in my arms (SP will have decreased reflexes in left arm).

___23.   tested reflexes in my legs (SP will have decreased reflexes in left leg).

___24.   tested my Babinski reflex by scratching soles of my feet (SP will have upgoing left toe and downgoing right toe).

___25.   listened to my heart in at least three places.

___26.   listened to my lungs in at least four places (normal lung examination).

Communication Skills. The Examinee:

___27.   made empathetic statements.

___28.   explained the diagnostic possibilities to me (i.e., stroke, transient ischemic attack, brain hemorrhage).

___29.   explained about hypertension as a risk factor for stroke.

___30.   explained the plan (blood work, electrocardiogram, CT scan of the head, neurology consultation, carotid ultrasound with Doppler, echocardiogram).

___31.   explained the treatment (admission to hospital, blood pressure control, perhaps fibrinolytics).

___32.   inquired about any family members who should be notified.

If you performed 23 of these 32 tasks, you passed this test station.

You have 10 minutes to complete your patient note.

HISTORY—Include significant positives and negatives from the history of present illness, past medical history, review of systems, and social and family history.

_____
_____
_____
_____
_____
_____
_____
_____
_____
_____
_____

PHYSICAL EXAMINATION—Indicate only the pertinent positive and negative findings related to the patient's chief complaint.

_____
_____
_____
_____
_____
_____
_____
_____
_____
_____
_____

DIFFERENTIAL DIAGNOSIS—In order of likelihood, write no more than five differential diagnoses for this patient's current problems.

1. _____
2. _____
3. _____
4. _____
5. _____

DIAGNOSTIC WORKUP—Immediate plans for no more than five diagnostic studies.

1. _____
2. _____
3. _____
4. _____
5. _____

A SATISFACTORY PATIENT NOTE

HISTORY—Include significant positives and negatives from the history of present illness, past medical history, review of systems, and social and family history.

Mrs. Eva Divine is a 73-year-old retired accountant who presents with a 4-hour history of left arm and leg weakness, which occurred suddenly while she was watching television. Her speech is not affected but she states that both her left arm and leg feel numb. She denies vision changes or headache, but when she looked in the mirror she noticed her face was twisted. She denies tobacco or alcohol use. Her past medical history is significant for hypertension controlled with diet and exercise. She has no history of diabetes. She denies chest pain, shortness of breath, palpitations, dizziness, an irregular heartbeat or syncope. She did not fall recently and denies head trauma.

PHYSICAL EXAMINATION—Indicate only the pertinent positive and negative findings related to the patient's chief complaint.

Patient is a well-developed, well-nourished female who is tearful and anxious.
BP = 170/110 mmHg right arm and 175/110 mmHg left arm. HR 86 and regular. RR 14. Speech is fluent.
HEENT: Facial asymmetry. Shallow left nasolabial fold. PERLA. EOMI. No JVD. No carotid bruits. Fundi normal. No visual field deficits. Tongue deviates to the left.
Heart: Normal S_1 and S_2. No gallops, rubs, or murmurs.
Lungs: Clear to auscultation and percussion.
Neuro: Alert, oriented × 3. CN II-XII normal except for left 7th CN.
Motor: Strength RUE and RLE is 5/5. Strength 3/5 LUE and LLE.
Sensory: Normal dull-sharp RUE and RLE. Decreased dull-sharp LUE and LLE.
DTR: 2+ Right brachial, triceps, patellar, and achilles.
1+ Left brachial, triceps, patellar, and achilles.
Positive left-sided Babinski reflex.

DIFFERENTIAL DIAGNOSIS
In order of likelihood, write no more than five differential diagnoses for this patient's current problems.

1. cerebrovascular accident (CVA)
2. transient ischemic attack (TIA)
3. subdural hematoma
4. intracranial hemorrhage
5. intracranial mass

DIAGNOSTIC WORKUP
Immediate plans for no more than five diagnostic studies.

1. CT scan of the head
2. electrocardiogram
3. echocardiogram
4. carotid Dopplers
5.

LEARNING OBJECTIVE FOR MRS. DIVINE
RECOGNIZE A TRANSIENT ISCHEMIC ATTACK OR EARLY STROKE

Risk factors for thrombotic stroke include hypertension, tobacco use, drug use, excessive alcohol use, diabetes mellitus, and hyperlipidemia. Atrial fibrillation and valvular heart disease are risk factors for embolic stroke. Mrs. Divine presents with a neurologic deficit and is hypertensive. She had no cardiac complaints. A history of frequent falls from either alcohol use or aging is denied by Mrs. Divine. She has no history of recent head trauma. The physical examination reveals no evidence of congestive heart failure. The neurologic examination reveals normal-sized, reactive pupils and weak left upper and lower extremities. Mrs. Divine has a hemisensory loss and is hyporeflexic, with a positive Babinski reflex on the affected extremity. There is facial asymmetry (shallow left nasolabial fold) and left facial weakness, but her speech is fluent. The tongue deviates to the left side. Auscultation of the carotid arteries reveals no audible bruit. The presentation is consistent with a right (nondominant) acute hemispheric stroke.

The workup for Mrs. Divine requires cardiac and neurologic evaluations. Thrombolytic agents will be considered for her stroke if hemorrhage is ruled out by CT scan of the head and blood pressure is controlled. Atrial fibrillation is a risk factor for embolic stroke and Mrs. Divine will need an electrocardiogram and perhaps an echocardiogram to look for thrombus.

Patient Note Pearl: The **differential diagnosis** for this patient with left-sided weakness includes stroke (thrombotic or embolic), hemorrhage, transient ischemic attack, subdural hematoma, intracranial mass, and hypoglycemia. The **diagnostic workup** for this patient would include a serum glucose level, serum lipid profile, a CT scan of the head, electrocardiogram, echocardiogram (looking for thrombus formation), and carotid Doppler studies.

Case 13

Your golfing buddy, a dermatologist, asks you to consult on a 25-year-old female law student named Judy Justice. She originally presented to the dermatology practice complaining of a 1-month history of leg rash, which your friend immediately biopsied. The skin biopsy revealed discoid lupus. The rash resolved after a 2-week course of hydrocortisone cream.

Vital Signs:

Temperature	98.6°F
Blood pressure	110/70 mmHg
Heart rate	72 beats per minute
Respiratory rate	12 breaths per minute

Upon entering the examination room, you notice a smiling young woman dressed in a T-shirt and shorts, wearing a scarf on her head.

Examinee's Tasks

1. Obtain a focused and relevant history.
2. Perform a focused and relevant physical examination.
3. Discuss your initial diagnostic impressions with the patient.
4. Discuss follow-up tests with the patient.
5. After seeing the patient, complete paperwork relevant to the case.

MY CHECKLIST

History of Present Illness. The Examinee:

1. _____
2. _____
3. _____
4. _____
5. _____
6. _____
   _____
7. _____
8. _____
9. _____
10. _____
11. _____
    _____
12. _____
13. _____
14. _____
15. _____

Physical Examination. The Examinee:

16. _____
    _____
17. _____
18. _____
19. _____
20. _____

Communication Skills. The Examinee:

21. _____
22. _____
23. _____
    _____
24. _____
25. _____
26. _____
27. _____
28. _____

SP CHECKLIST ON MS. JUSTICE

History of Present Illness. The Examinee:

___ 1. asked about any hair loss ("It comes out in chunks in the shower; I have to wear this scarf to hide bald spots.")

___ 2. asked about any joint pain ("For the last month, my wrists and fingers have been painful and stiff.")

___ 3. asked about photosensitivity, i.e., if sun causes skin color changes ("Yes.")

___ 4. asked about other rashes ("Yes. Once I had a facial rash; it was in a butterfly pattern.")

___ 5. asked about oral ulcers ("Yes. My roommate thought they were from stress.")

___ 6. asked about generalized symptoms, i.e., fever, malaise, weight loss ("Yes, I have lost 8 pounds, and I often have a temperature of 100.4°F, and I am always tired.")

___ 7. asked about heart symptoms, i.e., chest pain, palpitations ("No.")

___ 8. asked about pulmonary complaints, i.e., shortness of breath, cough ("No.")

___ 9. asked about neurologic complaints, i.e., seizures, weakness, numbness ("No.")

___10. asked about urinary problems, i.e., hematuria, foamy urine ("No.")

___11. asked about cold temperature causing problems with my fingers, i.e., Raynaud's phenomenon ("Sometimes my fingers become pale and then blue when I go outside in the cold weather.")

___12. asked about a history of pregnancy, i.e., miscarriages ("No.")

___13. asked about medications ("None.")

___14. asked about alcohol, tobacco, and drug use ("None of those things.")

___15. asked about a family history of collagen vascular disease ("I had a cousin who died from lupus.")

Physical Examination. The Examinee:

___16. asked me to remove my scarf to examine my scalp for alopecia, i.e., hair loss (SP has numerous bald spots when scarf is removed).

___17. looked in my mouth for ulcers (none are seen).

___18. checked at least three joints for any abnormalities (no joint tenderness or warmth; no nodules).

___19. listened to my heart (normal examination).

___20. listened to my lungs (normal examination).

Communication Skills. The Examinee:

___21. introduced self to me.

___22. put me at ease.

___23. gave me information about the diagnostic possibilities [systemic lupus erythematosus (SLE) or other collagen vascular disease].

___24. talked about the plan in an organized fashion (blood work, urinalysis, immunologic markers).

___25. checked my understanding of the problem.

___26. offered me continuous and ongoing support.

___27. discussed a follow-up appointment with me.

___28. when I expressed concern about my career choice, stated that I could still be a lawyer.

If you performed 20 of these 28 tasks, you passed this test station.

You have 10 minutes to complete your patient note.

HISTORY—Include significant positives and negatives from the history of present illness, past medical history, review of systems, and social and family history.

_____
_____
_____
_____
_____
_____
_____
_____
_____
_____
_____

PHYSICAL EXAMINATION—Indicate only the pertinent positive and negative findings related to the patient's chief complaint.

_____
_____
_____
_____
_____
_____
_____
_____
_____
_____
_____

DIFFERENTIAL DIAGNOSIS—In order of likelihood, write no more than five differential diagnoses for this patient's current problems.

1. _____
2. _____
3. _____
4. _____
5. _____

DIAGNOSTIC WORKUP—Immediate plans for no more than five diagnostic studies.

1. _____
2. _____
3. _____
4. _____
5. _____

A SATISFACTORY PATIENT NOTE

HISTORY—Include significant positives and negatives from the history of present illness, past medical history, review of systems, and social and family history.

Ms. Judy Justice is a 25-year-old law student who is referred by a dermatologist after a biopsy of a leg rash revealed discoid lupus. The patient developed the rash 1 month prior to the biopsy. Ms. Justice states that previous to this rash she developed an erythematous facial rash that was in a butterfly pattern over her cheeks and nose. She did not seek medical attention for the rash and it resolved after a month. The patient also admits to previously having oral ulcers and photosensitivity. At times, she has painful and stiff wrist and finger joints and generalized fatigue. She has lost 8 pounds and has had temperatures to 100.4°F. Her fingers often become pale and blue in cold weather. Additionally, she has been noticing that her hair is falling out in chunks and she is developing areas of baldness requiring her to wear a scarf. She denies chest pain, shortness of breath, palpitations, and cough. She denies neurological complaints, such as seizures, weakness and numbness. She has no urinary problems, such as hematuria or foamy urine. She has never been pregnant and has had no miscarriages. She does not smoke, drink, or use illicit drugs. Family history is remarkable for a cousin who died of systemic lupus erythematosus. She takes no medications.

PHYSICAL EXAMINATION—Indicate only the pertinent positive and negative findings related to the patient's chief complaint.

Vital signs are normal. The patient is a well-developed, well-nourished young woman who is pleasant and cooperative.
Skin: No malar rash. No nodules.
HEENT: Positive for alopecia. No oral ulcers.
Lungs: clear to auscultation and percussion.
Heart: Normal S_1 and S_2. No murmurs, rubs, or gallops.
Abdomen: Normal BS. Nontender.
Extremities: No joint warmth, erythema, deformities or tenderness.
Neuro: Alert 0×3. No focal abnormalities.

DIFFERENTIAL DIAGNOSIS

In order of likelihood, write no more than five differential diagnoses for this patient's current problems.

1. SLE
2. discoid lupus
3. progressive systemic sclerosis
4. rheumatoid arthritis
5.

DIAGNOSTIC WORKUP

Immediate plans for no more than five diagnostic studies.

1. CBC
2. electrolytes
3. urinalysis
4. ANA
5. Anti–double-stranded DNA

LEARNING OBJECTIVE FOR MS. JUSTICE
RECOGNIZE THE VARIABLE SYMPTOMATOLOGY OF
THE COLLAGEN VASCULAR DISEASE

Ms. Judy Justice has recently been diagnosed with discoid lupus. The dermatologist has now referred the patient to you for further investigation of her symptoms.

Initially, Ms. Justice tells you she has no complaints. The plaque on her leg that was biopsied has resolved with the steroid cream prescribed by the dermatologist. As the physician begins to investigate systemic involvement in this patient, it becomes plausible that Ms. Justice may have SLE. The risk factors for SLE include a genetic predisposition, and Ms. Justice admits that a cousin died of lupus. Most cases of the disease occur in women during their childbearing years, and Ms. Justice is 25 years old. Drugs may induce lupus, but the patient does not take any medications such as isoniazid, hydralazine, or procainamide.

Ms. Justice admits to having several symptoms of SLE including joint pain, Raynaud's phenomenon, hair loss, malar rash, and photosensitivity. She also complains of weight loss, fever, and generalized malaise. She has no heart, lung, kidney, or central nervous system complaints. She has no previous history of miscarriages, which may be seen in SLE patients with antiphospholipid antibodies.

Heart and lung examinations reveal no evidence of pericarditis or pleuritis. Ulcers are not present in the mouth and the joints are normal. Alopecia is evident after the patient is asked to remove her scarf and the scalp is examined.

The differential diagnosis for Ms. Justice should include autoimmune diseases such as SLE, rheumatoid arthritis, and progressive systemic sclerosis. Further evaluation looking for hematologic abnormalities (thrombocytopenia, anemia, leukopenia), renal dysfunction (hematuria and proteinuria), and immunologic markers is required.

Ms. Justice requires reassurance that the outlook for patients with this disease has improved significantly and that, with proper treatment, she can continue her studies and become a lawyer.

Patient Note Pearl: The **differential diagnosis** for this patient may include SLE, discoid lupus, progressive systemic sclerosis, and rheumatoid arthritis. The **diagnostic workup** may include CBC with platelet count, electrolytes, urinalysis, the antinuclear antibody test, and antibodies to double-stranded DNA.

NOTES

Case 14

A 65-year-old man named Charlie Champion presents to your office complaining of difficulty swallowing.

Vital Signs:

Temperature	98.6°F
Blood pressure	100/70 mmHg
Heart rate	88 beats per minute
Respiratory rate	12 breaths per minute

Examinee's Tasks

1. Obtain a focused and relevant history.
2. Perform a focused and relevant physical examination.
3. Discuss initial diagnostic impressions with the patient.
4. Discuss follow-up tests with the patient.
5. After seeing the patient, complete paperwork relevant to the case.

MY CHECKLIST

History of Present Illness. The Examinee:

1. _____
   _____
2. _____
3. _____
4. _____
   _____
5. _____
6. _____
7. _____
   _____
8. _____
9. _____
10. _____
11. _____

Physical Examination. The Examinee:

12. _____
13. _____
14. _____

Communication Skills. The Examinee:

15. _____
16. _____
17. _____
   _____
18. _____
19. _____
20. _____
21. _____
22. _____
23. _____
24. _____

SP CHECKLIST FOR MR. CHAMPION

History of Present Illness. The Examinee:

___ 1. asked if there was "real dysphagia," i.e., a feeling of food sticking in the chest ("Yes, that describes what I'm feeling.")

___ 2. asked about the onset of dysphagia ("It started about 2 months ago.")

___ 3. asked specifically about difficulty swallowing solid foods ("I definitely can't swallow anything solid.")

___ 4. asked specifically about difficulty swallowing liquids ("Not in the beginning, but now it's getting to the point where swallowing water is becoming a problem.")

___ 5. asked about painful swallowing, i.e., odynophagia ("No.")

___ 6. asked about weight loss ("Yes. I've lost 20 pounds in the last month.")

___ 7. asked about alcohol use ("I used to be a heavy drinker—a pint of whiskey a day for 25 years; I stopped drinking 2 months ago, when this problem started.")

___ 8. asked about tobacco use ("Yes. I've smoked two packs of cigarettes per day for over 25 years.")

___ 9. asked about a previous history of gastrointestinal problems, i.e., reflux ("No.")

___10. asked about a history of lye ingestion ("No.")

___11. asked about any hoarseness ("No.")

Physical Examination. The Examinee:

___12. looked inside my mouth for obstructive lesions (normal mouth and pharynx).

___13. checked my neck for an enlarged thyroid gland or other obstructive masses (none evident).

___14. checked for either axillary or supraclavicular nodes (a 3-cm fixed left supraclavicular node is palpable).

Communication Skills. The Examinee:

___15. explained the possible diagnosis (esophageal carcinoma, achalasia, stricture).

___16. explained that risk factors for the disease include tobacco and alcohol use.

___17. explained the next step in the workup (blood work, esophagogram, gastroenterology consultation for possible endoscopy).

___18. explained that the supraclavicular node was probably due to cancer.

___19. stated that I would need nutritional support either in the hospital or at home.

___20. inquired about my support system ("I have a wife at home; no children.")

___21. offered to help me tell my wife ("Oh, that would be a big help, Doctor.")

___22. demonstrated empathy for my situation.

___23. discussed prognosis (this is a serious problem).

___24. asked me if there was anything not covered in the discussion.

If you performed 17 of these 24 tasks, you passed this test station.

You have 10 minutes to complete your patient note.

HISTORY—Include significant positives and negatives from the history of present illness, past medical history, review of systems, and social and family history.

_____
_____
_____
_____
_____
_____
_____
_____
_____
_____

PHYSICAL EXAMINATION—Indicate only the pertinent positive and negative findings related to the patient's chief complaint.

_____
_____
_____
_____
_____
_____
_____
_____
_____
_____

DIFFERENTIAL DIAGNOSIS—In order of likelihood, write no more than five differential diagnoses for this patient's current problems.

1. _____
2. _____
3. _____
4. _____
5. _____

DIAGNOSTIC WORKUP—Immediate plans for no more than five diagnostic studies.

1. _____
2. _____
3. _____
4. _____
5. _____

A SATISFACTORY PATIENT NOTE

HISTORY—Include significant positives and negatives from the history of present illness, past medical history, review of systems, and social and family history.

Mr. Charlie Champion is a 65-year-old man with a 2-month history of dysphagia. He feels as if the food he eats is getting stuck in the middle of his chest. Two months ago, the dysphagia was occurring only with solids, but it has now progressed to liquids to the point where the patient is having difficulty swallowing water. Mr. Champion denies odynophagia but admits to a 20-pound weight loss over the last month. He is a former drinker of a pint of whiskey daily for 25 years but stopped 2 months ago. He has smoked 2 packs of cigarettes per day for over 25 years. He has no previous history of gastrointestinal problems, such as reflux, and has no history of lye ingestion. He denies hoarseness.

PHYSICAL EXAMINATION—Indicate only the pertinent positive and negative findings related to the patient's chief complaint.

Cachectic male looking older than his stated age in NAD. Patient is not hoarse. HT = 72 in. WT = 140 lb.
BP = 100/70 mmHg and HR = 88 beats/min lying down.
BP = 100/70 mmHg and HR = 88 beats/min standing.
Afebrile. RR = 12 breaths/min.
HEENT: Mouth without lesions or masses. Thyroid normal.
3-cm fixed nontender left supraclavicular node.
No cervical, submandibular, occipital, or submental lymphadenopathy. No axillary lymphadenopathy.
Heart, lungs, and **abdominal** exams normal.

DIFFERENTIAL DIAGNOSIS
In order of likelihood, write no more than five differential diagnoses for this patient's current problems.

1. esophageal carcinoma
2. stricture
3. achalasia
4. Schatzki's ring
5.

DIAGNOSTIC WORKUP
Immediate plans for no more than five diagnostic studies.

1. barium esophagogram
2. endoscopy with biopsy and histology
3. CBC
4. electrolytes
5. liver function tests

LEARNING OBJECTIVE FOR MR. CHAMPION
APPROACH TO THE PATIENT WITH DYSPHAGIA

Mr. Champion presents with the chief complaint of dysphagia, initially to solids then progressing to liquids (progressive dysphagia), accompanied by anorexia and rapid weight loss. It is important to inquire about the symptoms of dysphagia (food sticking implies real dysphagia). Dysphagia accompanied by odynophagia (painful swallowing) may indicate mediastinal invasion by tumor. Other symptoms of esophageal cancer may include cough, hoarseness, choking, fever, and aspiration pneumonitis. The patient has a long history of alcohol and tobacco abuse, which predisposes him to developing esophageal carcinoma. Other risk factors for esophageal cancer include chronic gastric reflux causing a Barrett's esophagus, achalasia, and lye ingestion. The differential diagnosis for dysphagia in this patient would include a stricture and achalasia.

On physical examination, Mr. Champion has a normal-sounding voice. Tumor involvement of the recurrent laryngeal nerve would cause hoarseness. The mouth and neck examinations reveal no obstructive lesions responsible for the dysphagia. A careful search for metastatic lymphadenopathy reveals a fixed node in the left supraclavicular area. In most cases, the physical examination in patients with esophageal carcinoma is unremarkable.

The workup for Mr. Champion includes admission to the hospital for nutritional support to prevent further weight loss. A barium esophagogram is the first step in the workup of any patient with dysphagia. If a lesion is seen radiographically, further evaluation with endoscopy, biopsy, and histologic assessment is warranted to confirm the diagnosis. Patients with poor nutritional intake should be evaluated with a complete blood count and electrolytes. Elevated liver function tests may be representative of metastasis to the liver.

The treatment for esophageal carcinoma is palliative when the disease is metastatic. The goal of therapy is to relieve the dysphagia if possible and maximize the quality of life for each patient.

Patient Note Pearl: The **differential diagnosis** for esophageal dysphagia is as follows:

Solid food dysphagia (mechanical problem)
    Intermittent: lower esophagus (Schatzki's ring)
    Progressive: stricture (has heartburn),
                 cancer

Solid or liquid dysphagia (neuromuscular problem)
    Intermittent: diffuse esophageal spasm (has chest pain)
    Progressive: scleroderma (has heartburn),
                 achalasia (may have respiratory symptoms)

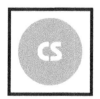

Case 15

A 62-year-old man, Samuel Samson, has an appointment to see you. His neighbor has scheduled the appointment for Mr. Samson because he has noticed that his friend, who is having difficulty walking, frequently trips and falls at home. The neighbor fears that one day Mr. Samson will really hurt himself.

Vital Signs:

Temperature	98.6°F
Blood pressure	160/80 mmHg
Heart rate	80 beats per minute and regular
Respiratory rate	12 breaths per minute

Upon entering the examination room, you see a man who looks older than his stated age. He is disheveled in appearance. He has noticeable tremors of his right hand.

Examinee's Tasks

1. Obtain a focused and relevant history.
2. Perform a focused and relevant physical examination.
3. Discuss your initial diagnostic impressions with the patient.
4. Discuss follow-up tests with the patient.
5. After seeing the patient, complete paperwork relevant to the case.

MY CHECKLIST

History of Present Illness. The Examinee:

1. _____
2. _____
3. _____
   _____
4. _____
5. _____
6. _____
7. _____
8. _____
9. _____
10. _____
    _____
11. _____
    _____

Physical Examination. The Examinee:

12. _____
13. _____
    _____
14. _____
15. _____
16. _____
17. _____
18. _____
19. _____
20. _____
21. _____
    _____

Communication Skills. The Examinee:

22. _____
23. _____
24. _____
25. _____
26. _____
27. _____
28. _____

SP CHECKLIST FOR MR. SAMSON

History of Present Illness. The Examinee:

___ 1. asked about the onset of difficulty walking ("It started about 3 months ago.")

___ 2. asked if the difficulty walking was progressively becoming worse ("Yes, it's getting worse; it's sure not any better.")

___ 3. asked if the difficulty walking is aggravated or precipitated by anything ("Yes, if I'm stressed about something, I seem to get worse.")

___ 4. asked about numbness and tingling of extremities ("No.")

___ 5. asked about the onset of tremors at rest ("Oh, these started maybe a year ago; aren't these due to old age?")

___ 6. asked about a family history of tremors ("No one in my family has these tremors.")

___ 7. asked about difficulty writing ("Yes, my signature doesn't even look like mine anymore.")

___ 8. asked about a family history of neurologic problems ("Nope.")

___ 9. asked about any medications ("None.")

___10. asked about the performance of other activities of daily living (ADLs) besides walking, i.e., bathing, feeding, toileting, dressing, transferring into and out of chairs and bed ("I sometimes have a little trouble getting out of chairs, I have a little trouble with buttons and zippers when I get dressed, and sometimes I don't make it to the bathroom; lately, I've been wearing a diaper when I go out.")

___11. asked about the performance of IADLs, i.e., shopping, traveling, cooking, managing money, using the telephone, and cleaning the house ("My good neighbor helps me with the bills, shopping, and cooking. The house is usually a mess, and I don't own a phone anymore.")

Physical Examination. The Examinee:

___12. checked the patient for cogwheel rigidity (SP will have cogwheel rigidity).

___13. asked the patient to perform a task to verify that tremor disappears with intention (SP will stop tremors with movement; tremors will occur at rest only).

___14. checked seventh cranial nerve, i.e., raise eyebrows, smile and blow out cheeks (normal).

___15. checked strength of upper extremity (normal).

___16. checked strength of lower extremity (normal).

___17. checked deep tendon reflexes in arm (normal).

___18. checked deep tendon reflexes in leg (normal).

___19. checked rapid alternating movements (slow due to rigidity).

___20. checked for Romberg (normal but torso tug is positive-moves in direction pushed).

___21. asked the patient to try to get out of a chair, walk across the room, turn around, and return to the chair (SP will have difficulty getting out of chair, gait will be shuffling, posture will be flexed and leaning forward, and small steps will be taken by the patient, with difficulty initiating and stopping ambulation; SP will turn en bloc; decreased arm swing when walking).

Communication Skills. The Examinee:

___22. explained my physical findings to me (tremors, gait, cogwheel rigidity).

___23. discussed the diagnostic possibilities with me (i.e., Parkinson's disease, hypothyroidism, dementia).

___24. discussed treatment (medications).

___25. discussed prognosis (some of the symptoms may improve with medication).

___26. discussed community resources that can help me to remain at home.

___27. offered ongoing support and help.

___28. scheduled follow-up appointment with me.

If you performed 20 of these 28 tasks, you passed this test station.

You have 10 minutes to complete your patient note.

HISTORY—Include significant positives and negatives from the history of present illness, past medical history, review of systems, and social and family history.

_____

_____

_____

_____

_____

_____

_____

_____

_____

_____

PHYSICAL EXAMINATION—Indicate only the pertinent positive and negative findings related to the patient's chief complaint.

_____

_____

_____

_____

_____

_____

_____

_____

_____

DIFFERENTIAL DIAGNOSIS—In order of likelihood, write no more than five differential diagnoses for this patient's current problems.

1. _____

2. _____

3. _____

4. _____

5. _____

DIAGNOSTIC WORKUP—Immediate plans for no more than five diagnostic studies.

1. _____

2. _____

3. _____

4. _____

5. _____

A SATISFACTORY PATIENT NOTE

HISTORY—Include significant positives and negatives from the history of present illness, past medical history, review of systems, and social and family history.

Mr. Samuel Samson is a 62-year-old man who has been having increasing difficulty walking over the last 3 months. He denies pain, numbness, and tingling of his extremities. He has a 1-year history of resting tremors, which he attributes to old age. His penmanship has deteriorated because of his tremors. He feels that stress makes the tremors and walking more difficult. He has trouble getting out of chairs and trouble with zippers and buttons when he tries to get dressed. He is having difficulty getting to the bathroom and is now wearing a diaper to prevent accidents when he leaves the house. His kindly neighbor helps him pay the bills and also with the shopping and cooking. He has no family history of tremors or of a neurologic disease. He takes no medications.

PHYSICAL EXAMINATION—Indicate only the pertinent positive and negative findings related to the patient's chief complaint.

Patient appears older than stated age of 62 years. Disheveled.
Walks with a shuffling gait, needing occasional support.
BP = 160/80 mmHg. HR = 82 beats/min. Afebrile. RR = 12 breaths/min.
HEENT: PERLA. EOMI. Minimal blinking and few facial movements.
Neuro: Alert. 0 × 3. CN II-XII intact.
Motor: Cogwheel rigidity. Strength normal.
Cerebellar: Normal rapid alternating movements but slow due to rigidity. Pill-rolling tremors at rest.
DTR: 2+ diffusely.
Romberg is normal. **Positive torso tug.**
Gait: Shuffling. Posture flexed and leaning forward. Difficulty initiating and stopping. Turns en bloc. Decreased arm swing.

DIFFERENTIAL DIAGNOSIS

In order of likelihood, write no more than five differential diagnoses for this patient's current problems.

1. Parkinson's disease
2. Wilson's disease
3. hypothyroidism
4. familial benign tremor
5.

DIAGNOSTIC WORKUP

Immediate plans for no more than five diagnostic studies.

1. trial with anti-Parkinson medication
2. TSH
3. ceruloplasmin
4.
5.

LEARNING OBJECTIVE FOR MR. SAMSON
FUNCTIONAL ASSESSMENT OF GAIT

This patient presents with resting tremors, bradykinesia, and a history of frequent falls. Mr. Samson's posture is flexed, and he has difficulty getting out of a chair due to his rigidity. He rarely blinks, has few facial movements, and walks without swinging his arms because of the paucity of his movements. His gait is shuffling (festinating) and consists of small steps. It is difficult for him to initiate and stop ambulation. For Mr. Samson, turning around when walking requires time and effort because of the many steps involved in this process. All of these symptoms are consistent with the diagnosis of Parkinson's disease.

On physical examination, Mr. Samson is found to have cogwheel rigidity. His right-hand pill-rolling tremors seem to worsen with stress and disappear with movement (if tested, he would also demonstrate micrographia). The MMSE result would be consistent with mild cognitive impairment. An assessment of his gait confirms that he is at risk for frequent falls due to the symptoms of Parkinson's disease.

With appropriate medications, such as anticholinergic or dopaminergic agents, Mr. Samson's symptoms may improve to the point where he can take better care of himself. For the time being, however, it is clear that the patient needs assistance at home. Mr. Samson has no family support system, but a caring neighbor seems to be interested in helping him. The neighbor, along with resources in the community, should be utilized to improve the quality of life that this patient has now. Careful follow-up of this patient would include home visits by a physician, nurse, and social worker.

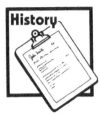

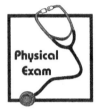

History-Taking Pearl: Elderly patients should be screened for frequent falls regardless of the presenting problem. Simply ask the patient if he or she has fallen all the way to the ground over the last 12 months. Measures to prevent falls include proper patient footwear and improved lighting in the home. Medications that contribute to falls in the elderly include sedatives, diuretics, and antidepressant agents.

Physical Examination Pearl: The "get up and go" test is an important assessment tool in elderly patients. The patient must get out of a chair, walk 10 ft, turn around, and walk back to the chair in less than 15 seconds. Gait abnormalities and the risk of falling can be assessed with this test. Individuals who perform poorly may benefit from physical therapy.

A patient with Parkinson's disease will remain stable during a Romberg test, but if pushed will move in the direction pushed (positive torso tug).

Patient Note Pearl: The **differential diagnosis** for this patient is Parkinson's disease, dementia, hypothyroidism, depression, essential familial (benign) tremor, parkinsonism due to postencephalitic illness, carbon monoxide poisoning, drugs (MPTP–a meperidine analogue used as an illicit drug, reserpine, metoclopramide, and neuroleptics), brain tumor, Huntington's chorea, and Wilson's disease. The diagnosis of Parkinson's disease is made by physical examination and the patient's good response to levodopa. **Laboratory tests** may include copper, ceruloplasmin, and TSH levels. A magnetic resonance imaging (MRI) scan is not helpful in diagnosing Parkinson's disease, and no biological marker exists to confirm the diagnosis. A therapeutic trial with an anti-Parkinson medication may be included as part of the workup.

NOTES

Case 16

An 18-year-old high school senior named Bruce Berger has made an urgent appointment to see you because of a headache that developed during football practice. He had to leave practice because of the severe pain.

Upon entering the room, you see a young man with eyes closed tightly holding the left side of his head.

Vital Signs:

Temperature	98.8°F
Blood pressure	110/75 mmHg
Heart rate	76 beats per minute
Respiratory rate	12 breaths per minute

Examinee's Tasks

1. Obtain a focused and relevant history.
2. Perform a focused and relevant physical examination.
3. Discuss your initial diagnostic impressions with the patient.
4. Discuss follow-up tests with the patient.
5. After seeing the patient, complete paperwork relevant to the case.

MY CHECKLIST

History of Present Illness. The Examinee:

1. _____
2. _____
3. _____
4. _____
5. _____
6. _____
7. _____
8. _____
9. _____
10. _____
11. _____
12. _____
    _____
13. _____
14. _____
15. _____
16. _____
17. _____

Physical Examination. The Examinee:

18. _____
19. _____
20. _____
21. _____
22. _____
23. _____
24. _____

Communication Skills. The Examinee:

25. _____
    _____
26. _____
27. _____
28. _____
29. _____
    _____
30. _____

SP CHECKLIST FOR MR. BERGER

History of Present Illness. The Examinee:

___ 1.   asked about the onset of the headache ("It started 3 hours ago after football practice.")

___ 2.   asked about the quality of the headache ("Pounding and throbbing.")

___ 3.   asked about progression of the headache ("It seems to be getting worse. It seems to be building up.")

___ 4.   asked about the location of the headache ("The entire left side of my head.")

___ 5.   asked about the intensity of the headache ("On a scale of 1 to 10, this is a 10.")

___ 6.   asked about alleviating factors ("Closing my eyes and staying very still help; I took 2 aspirin and they didn't help.")

___ 7.   asked about aggravating factors ("Movement, light, and noise make it worse.")

___ 8.   asked about any association with nausea or vomiting ("I vomited once and I still feel nauseated.")

___ 9.   asked about neurologic deficits, i.e., weakness, sensory changes, speech difficulties ("No.")

___10.   asked about an aura preceding headache ("Lights were flashing for about 20 minutes before it started.")

___11.   asked about recent fever ("No.")

___12.   asked about a previous history of headaches ("I suffer with bad headaches, but they usually go away in 2 hours. I've had headaches for 10 years.")

___13.   asked what precipitates the headaches ("The stress of exams or important football games.")

___14.   asked about a family history of headache ("My mother and sister have migraines.")

___15.   asked about a history of head trauma during football practice ("No.")

___16.   asked about illicit drug use ("No.")

___17.   asked about alcohol use ("No.")

Physical Examination. The Examinee:

___18.   evaluated pupillary response to light with a flashlight (normal examination of pupils).

___19.   looked into my eyes with an ophthalmoscope (normal funduscopic examination).

___20.   palpated my TM joint and asked me to open my mouth (no clicking or pain).

___21.   palpated over my sinuses for tenderness (no tenderness).

___22.   evaluated my neck for stiffness (no nuchal rigidity).

___23.   tested the reflexes in my arms or legs (normal reflexes).

___24.   tested the muscle strength in my arms or legs (normal strength).

Communication Skills. The Examinee:

___25.   discussed the initial impression with me (diagnostic possibilities include migraine, cluster headache, and tension headache).

___26.   discussed the plan with me (medication).

___27.   discussed how the stress of football practice may have precipitated the headache.

___28.   explained that my family history of migraine headaches places me at risk for migraine headaches.

___29.   discussed other precipitating factors for migraine headaches (alcohol use, chocolate, monosodium glutamate, hunger, lack of sleep).

___30.   acknowledged my distress and discomfort.

If you performed 22 of these 30 tasks, you passed this test station.

You have 10 minutes to complete your patient note.

HISTORY—Include significant positives and negatives from the history of present illness, past medical history, review of systems, and social and family history.

_____

_____

_____

_____

_____

_____

_____

_____

_____

_____

_____

PHYSICAL EXAMINATION—Indicate only the pertinent positive and negative findings related to the patient's chief complaint.

_____

_____

_____

_____

_____

_____

_____

_____

_____

_____

_____

DIFFERENTIAL DIAGNOSIS—In order of likelihood, write no more than five differential diagnoses for this patient's current problems.

1. _____

2. _____

3. _____

4. _____

5. _____

DIAGNOSTIC WORKUP—Immediate plans for no more than five diagnostic studies.

1. _____

2. _____

3. _____

4. _____

5. _____

A SATISFACTORY PATIENT NOTE

HISTORY—Include significant positives and negatives from the history of present illness, past medical history, review of systems, and social and family history.

Mr. Bruce Berger is an 18-year old high school senior who presents with a 3-hour history of left-sided headache. The headache was preceded by 20 minutes of flashing lights and is pounding and throbbing in nature. The pain has progressively been getting worse and on a scale of 1 to 10 is a 10. The headache is aggravated by movement, light, and noise and is alleviated with lying still and closing the eyes. The headache is accompanied by nausea and vomiting. The patient denies any fever, sensory deficits, weakness, or speech difficulties. He took 2 aspirin with no relief. Mr. Berger has a 10-year history of headaches, which are brought on by stressful situations such as exams or important football games. He states that this headache began at football practice for the big game coming up but denies head trauma. He has a family history of migraines. He does not drink alcohol or use illicit drugs.

PHYSICAL EXAMINATION—Indicate only the pertinent positive and negative findings related to the patient's chief complaint.

T = 98.8°F. BP = 110/75 mmHg. HR = 76 beats/min. RR = 12 breaths/min.
The patient is a well-developed, well-nourished male sitting with eyes closed and holding the left side of his head. He appears to be in severe pain.
HEENT: PERLA. EOMI. Fundi benign. + Photophobia. No neck rigidity. TMJ joint opens normally without pain or click. No sinus tenderness.
Neuro: Alert and oriented × 3.
Cranial Nerves II-XII intact.
Normal muscle strength.
DTR 2+ diffusely.

DIFFERENTIAL DIAGNOSIS	**DIAGNOSTIC WORKUP**
In order of likelihood, write no more than five differential diagnoses for this patient's current problems.	Immediate plans for no more than five diagnostic studies.
1. migraine headache	1. CT scan of the head
2. tension headache	2.
3. cluster headache	3.
4. subdural hematoma	4.
5. subarachnoid hemorrhage	5.

LEARNING OBJECTIVE FOR MR. BERGER
APPROACH TO THE PATIENT WHO PRESENTS WITH HEADACHE

Mr. Berger has a presentation consistent with "classic" migraine headaches. He has a severe, throbbing, left-sided headache associated with vomiting and aggravated by bright light or noise. A 20-minute aura of flashing lights preceded the headache. He had to interrupt his activities because of the intensity of the headache. He has a 10-year history of headaches (migraines may start around the time of puberty) and a family history remarkable for migraines. He feels that this headache was precipitated by the stress of the big football game scheduled for the weekend.

Mr. Berger denies having any recent fever or illness that might suggest an infectious etiology for his headaches (sinusitis or meningitis). He has neither sinus tenderness nor neck rigidity. Subarachnoid hemorrhage must be considered in the differential diagnosis for this patient, but he has a long history of similar headaches and has no changes in his neurologic status. The patient denies having risk factors for stroke, such as cocaine use. Subdural hematoma (especially since the headache started during football practice) is unlikely without a history of head trauma. Temporal arteritis is uncommon in an 18-year-old man. Tension headaches are usually described as being band-like and occipital in location. Cluster headaches are brief frontal headaches often associated with tearing and nasal stuffiness.

Migraine headaches may be precipitated by diet (cheese, chocolate, processed meats), stress, menses, lack of sleep, exercise, sexual intercourse, hunger, and alcoholic beverages (the patient denies alcohol use). "Common" migraine (without aura) lacks neurologic symptoms, while "classic" (with aura) and "complicated" migraines may present with focal neurologic deficits. Common migraines are five times more common than classic migraines. Serotonin agonists and ergotamine agents act by vasoconstricting cranial blood vessels and are used to treat acute episodes of migraine. Patients who have frequent migraine attacks require prophylactic therapy.

History-Taking Pearl: Remember the **POUND**ing headaches mnemonic for migraine: **P** = **p**ulsating; **O** = last **o**ne day; **U** = **u**nilateral; **N** = associated with **n**ausea; **D** = **d**isturbance in daily activities; if the patient answers yes to four of these questions, it is most likely a migraine headache.

Patient Note Pearl: The **differential diagnosis** for headache includes migraine headache, tension headache, cluster headache, subdural hematoma, sinus headache, TMJ disease, meningitis, depression, subarachnoid hemorrhage, hypertension, intracranial mass, and temporal arteritis (palpate the temporal artery in older patients with headache). The **workup** may include a CBC, sedimentation rate, CT scan of the head, or an MRI scan when clinically indicated.

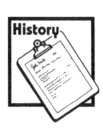

Case 17

An 18-year-old college freshman named Suzy Sunshine presents to the campus health center complaining of burning on urination. She is G0P0, menarche at age 13, with regular periods. Pelvic examination done by the nurse practitioner reveals no adnexal or cervical motion tenderness. There is no vaginal discharge.

Vital Signs:

Temperature	101.2°F
Blood pressure	105/70 mmHg
Heart rate	102 beats per minute
Respiratory rate	14 breaths per minute

Examinee's Tasks
(Do Not Repeat Gynecologic Examination)

1. Obtain a focused and relevant history.
2. Perform a focused and relevant physical examination.
3. Discuss your initial diagnostic impressions with the patient.
4. Discuss follow-up tests with the patient.
5. After seeing the patient, complete paperwork relevant to the case.

MY CHECKLIST

History of Present Illness. The Examinee:

1. _____
2. _____
3. _____
4. _____
5. _____
6. _____
7. _____
8. _____
9. _____
10. _____
11. _____
12. _____
13. _____

Physical Examination. The Examinee:

14. _____
15. _____
16. _____
17. _____

Communication Skills. The Examinee:

18. _____
19. _____
20. _____
21. _____
22. _____
23. _____
24. _____

SP CHECKLIST FOR MS. SUNSHINE

History of Present Illness. The Examinee:

___ 1. asked about the onset of dysuria ("It started 2 days ago.")

___ 2. asked about frequency of urination ("Yes, I urinate maybe 20 times a day.")

___ 3. asked about hematuria ("No.")

___ 4. asked about fever at home ("It was 101.5°F last night.")

___ 5. asked about shaking chills ("No.")

___ 6. asked about abdominal pain ("Yes, the lower part of my abdomen has been constantly hurting me.")

___ 7. asked about back pain ("Yes; the left side of my back hurts.")

___ 8. asked about nausea or vomiting ("No.")

___ 9. asked about diarrhea ("No.")

___10. asked about a history of urinary tract problems, i.e., stones, recurrent infections ("No.")

___11. asked about my last menstrual flow ("5 days ago; no problems.")

___12. asked about the possibility of pregnancy ("No. I have one partner, who uses condoms.")

___13. asked about a history of sexually transmitted diseases ("Never.")

Physical Examination. The Examinee:

___14. listened to my abdomen with a stethoscope (normal bowel sounds appreciated).

___15. pressed throughout my abdomen gently (no tenderness with mild palpation).

___16. pressed deeply throughout the abdomen (positive suprapubic tenderness with deep palpation).

___17. tapped on my back to elicit costovertebral angle tenderness (positive left costovertebral angle tenderness).

Communication Skills. The Examinee:

___18. washed hands before starting the physical examination.

___19. cared about my embarrassment during the physical examination.

___20. allowed me to dress fully before beginning discussion of my problem.

___21. discussed the diagnostic possibilities with me (i.e., pyelonephritis, kidney stone).

___22. discussed the workup in terms I could understand (urinalysis, urine culture, blood work).

___23. discussed the treatment with me (hydration, antibiotics).

___24. discussed the importance of close follow-up.

If you performed 17 of these 24 tasks, you passed this test station.

You have 10 minutes to complete your patient note.

HISTORY—Include significant positives and negatives from the history of present illness, past medical history, review of systems, and social and family history.

_____

_____

_____

_____

_____

_____

_____

_____

_____

_____

PHYSICAL EXAMINATION—Indicate only the pertinent positive and negative findings related to the patient's chief complaint.

_____

_____

_____

_____

_____

_____

_____

_____

_____

_____

DIFFERENTIAL DIAGNOSIS—In order of likelihood, write no more than five differential diagnoses for this patient's current problems.

1. _____

2. _____

3. _____

4. _____

5. _____

DIAGNOSTIC WORKUP—Immediate plans for no more than five diagnostic studies.

1. _____

2. _____

3. _____

4. _____

5. _____

A SATISFACTORY PATIENT NOTE

HISTORY—Include significant positives and negatives from the history of present illness, past medical history, review of systems, and social and family history.

Ms. Suzy Sunshine is an 18-year-old college student who presents with a 2-day history of burning on urination. She has had frequency up to 20 times a day and fever to 101.5°F. She denies hematuria and shaking chills. She has constant lower abdominal pain and left-sided back pain. She denies nausea, vomiting, and diarrhea. She has no past history of kidney stones or urinary tract infections. She has one sexual partner and always uses barrier protection. She has no vaginal discharge and has no history of sexually transmitted disease. Her LMP was 5 days ago and was normal. She had menarche at age 13, has regular periods, and is G0P0.

PHYSICAL EXAMINATION—Indicate only the pertinent positive and negative findings related to the patient's chief complaint.

Well-developed, well-nourished young woman in mild distress.
T = 101.2°F. HR = 102 beats/min. BP = 105/70 mmHg.
Lungs: Clear to auscultation.
Heart: Normal S_1 and S_2.
Abdomen: Normal BS. Positive suprapubic tenderness.
No guarding, rigidity or rebound. No masses.
Positive left CVA tenderness.
Pelvic: No discharge. No cervical motion tenderness. No adnexal tenderness.

DIFFERENTIAL DIAGNOSIS
In order of likelihood, write no more than five differential diagnoses for this patient's current problems.

1. pyelonephritis
2. kidney stone
3. cystitis
4.
5.

DIAGNOSTIC WORKUP
Immediate plans for no more than five diagnostic studies.

1. urinalysis
2. urine culture
3. urine Gram stain
4. CBC with differential
5. pregnancy test

LEARNING OBJECTIVE FOR MS. SUNSHINE
APPROACH TO THE PATIENT WITH DYSURIA

Ms. Suzy Sunshine presents with the complaints of fever, back pain, dysuria, and frequency. She denies having hematuria. She has no gynecologic or gastrointestinal complaints. Pelvic examination is normal. She has no previous history of urinary tract infection. She is not pregnant and has no history of previous sexually transmitted disease.

On physical examination, the patient has suprapubic tenderness on palpation and left costovertebral angle tenderness. The most likely diagnosis is pyelonephritis. The symptoms may include fever, abdominal pain, back or flank pain, nausea, vomiting, and diarrhea. Blood analysis will reveal a leukocytosis and urinalysis will be positive for nitrites, leukocytes, and bacteria.

Although most patients with pyelonephritis require hospitalization, this patient could probably be treated and managed as an outpatient. She is able to tolerate oral hydration and medications and will be compliant with a 14-day treatment regimen. She appears well and has no predisposing risk factor for infection (stones). Ms. Sunshine will be closely followed by her physician.

Patient Note Pearl: The **differential diagnosis** for this patient includes pyelonephritis and kidney stone. In any patient presenting with flank pain and fever, other etiologies should be considered, such as pneumonia, appendicitis, cholecystitis, pancreatitis, and diverticulitis. In this patient, these etiologies seem unlikely. The **workup** for this patient should include a CBC, urinalysis, urine Gram stain, and urine culture. Males with dysuria should be investigated for prostatitis and epididymitis.

Case 18

Eighteen-year-old Morgan Montgomery presents with a complaint of a rash. Upon entering the examination room, you see a young man with a circular lesion 15 cm in diameter located over his right lateral chest. The rash has a thin red border with central clearing.

Vital Signs:

Temperature	99.2°F
Blood pressure	115/75 mmHg
Heart rate	82 beats per minute
Respiratory rate	14 breaths per minute

Examinee's Tasks

1. Obtain a focused and relevant history.
2. Perform a focused and relevant physical examination.
3. Discuss your initial diagnostic impressions with the patient.
4. Discuss follow-up tests with the patient.
5. After seeing the patient, complete paperwork relevant to the case.

MY CHECKLIST

History of Present Illness. The Examinee:

1. _____
2. _____
3. _____
4. _____
5. _____
6. _____
7. _____
8. _____
9. _____
10. _____
11. _____
    _____
12. _____
13. _____
    _____
14. _____

Physical Examination. The Examinee:

15. _____
16. _____
    _____
17. _____
18. _____
19. _____
20. _____

Communication Skills. The Examinee:

21. _____
    _____
22. _____
23. _____
24. _____
25. _____

SP CHECKLIST FOR MR. MONTGOMERY

History of Present Illness. The Examinee:

___ 1. asked about the onset of the rash ("It started about 2 weeks ago; I thought it would go away.")

___ 2. asked if the rash was progressing ("Yes, it's getting wider with each day that goes by.")

___ 3. asked if the rash was pruritic ("No.")

___ 4. asked about recent insect bites ("None that I can remember.")

___ 5. asked about outdoor activity, e.g., camping or hiking ("No.")

___ 6. asked about occupation ("I'm a landscaper.")

___ 7. asked about fever ("Sometimes my temperature is 101°F.")

___ 8. asked about shaking chills ("Yes.")

___ 9. asked about muscle aches ("Yes.")

___10. asked about fatigue ("I have no energy; I am not feeling well. I'm tired all the time.")

___11. asked about headache ("Definitely. Intermittent, back part of head, and relieved with Tylenol. I never get headaches.")

___12. asked about any cardiac symptoms, e.g., palpitations, shortness of breath, chest pain ("No.")

___13. asked about any neurologic problems, e.g., stiff neck, numbness, vision changes, problems with gait or coordination ("No.")

___14. asked about joint pain ("No.")

Physical Examination. The Examinee:

___15. examined the rash closely (rash is warm and nontender).

___16. checked for lymphadenopathy, i.e., neck and axillary (few scattered, nontender, freely movable nodes are palpable in cervical and axillary areas).

___17. listened to my heart in at least three places (normal examination).

___18. checked at least two joints for abnormalities (normal joint examination).

___19. checked the movement of my eye muscles (normal extraocular muscle movement).

___20. checked sensation in my legs, i.e., sharp and dull, vibration (normal sensation).

Communication Skills. The Examinee:

___21. explained the initial impression (plausible diagnoses include Lyme disease, chronic fatigue syndrome, fibromyalgia).

___22. explained that a tick bite from my occupational exposure may have caused the rash.

___23. discussed the workup (blood work, electrocardiogram, frequent follow-up).

___24. explained that antibiotics would be needed if the problem was Lyme disease.

___25. answered all my questions in a manner I could understand.

If you performed 18 of these 25 tasks, you passed this test station.

You have 10 minutes to complete your patient note.

HISTORY—Include significant positives and negatives from the history of present illness, past medical history, review of systems, and social and family history.

_____
_____
_____
_____
_____
_____
_____
_____
_____
_____

PHYSICAL EXAMINATION—Indicate only the pertinent positive and negative findings related to the patient's chief complaint.

_____
_____
_____
_____
_____
_____
_____
_____
_____
_____

DIFFERENTIAL DIAGNOSIS—In order of likelihood, write no more than five differential diagnoses for this patient's current problems.

1. _____
2. _____
3. _____
4. _____
5 _____

DIAGNOSTIC WORKUP—Immediate plans for no more than five diagnostic studies.

1. _____
2. _____
3. _____
4. _____
5. _____

A SATISFACTORY PATIENT NOTE

HISTORY—Include significant positives and negatives from the history of present illness, past medical history, review of systems, and social and family history.

Mr. Morgan Montgomery is an 18-year-old landscaper who presents with a 2-week history of a 15-cm circular rash located on the lateral aspect of his right chest. He feels that the rash is getting wider as the days go by. He denies pruritus but has temperatures as high as 101.0°F accompanied by shaking chills. He does not recall any insect bites and has not recently gone camping or hiking. He does, however, work outdoors as a landscaper. He has generalized fatigue and has constant muscle aches. He has had intermittent occipital headaches that are relieved with Tylenol. He does not usually suffer from headaches. He denies chest pain, palpitations, shortness of breath, stiff neck, numbness, vision changes, and difficulties with gait or coordination. He has no joint pain.

PHYSICAL EXAMINATION—Indicate only the pertinent positive and negative findings related to the patient's chief complaint.

The patient is a well-developed, well-nourished young man who appears concerned but is in NAD. T = 99.2°F.
Right lateral chest: 15-cm rash that has a thin red border with central clearing. Rash is warm and nontender. No other rashes over body.
HEENT: PERLA. EOMI. No cervical or axillary lymphadenopathy.
Lungs: Clear to auscultation.
Heart: Normal S_1 and S_2. No rub is audible.
Extremities: No joint warmth, erythema, tenderness or deformities.
Neuro: CNII, V and VII intact. Normal sensation to touch.
Gait: Normal.

DIFFERENTIAL DIAGNOSIS

In order of likelihood, write no more than five differential diagnoses for this patient's current problems.

1. Lyme disease
2. chronic fatigue syndrome
3. fibromyalgia
4.
5.

DIAGNOSTIC WORKUP

Immediate plans for no more than five diagnostic studies.

1. ELISA for Lyme disease
2. Western blot test for Lyme disease
3. electrocardiogram
4.
5.

LEARNING OBJECTIVE FOR MR. MONTGOMERY
RECOGNIZE THAT A RASH CAN BE A SIGN OF SYSTEMIC DISEASE

Mr. Montgomery works as a landscaper and is at risk for tick-borne illness. He presents with erythema migrans (EM), the rash characteristic of Lyme disease. Lyme disease occurs mostly in the summer months and is caused by the spirochete *Borrelia burgdorferi*. It is important to obtain the appropriate history and perform a physical examination to determine the extent and stage of disease (localized or disseminated).

On questioning, Mr. Montgomery admits to having a headache, fever, chills, myalgias, and fatigue (this is often referred to as the *pentad* of Lyme disease). He denies having any cardiac, neurologic, or rheumatologic complaints. His heart examination reveals no evidence of pericarditis or left ventricular dysfunction (an electrocardiogram will be needed to exclude atrioventricular block). His rheumatologic examination reveals no joint warmth or erythema. On neurologic examination, cranial nerves and sensation are intact. There is no evidence of neuropathy or neuritis.

Lyme disease is a three-stage disease. **Stage one** disease (up to 20 days after the tick bite) consists of the classic lesion of EM (occurs in 70 percent of patients) and flu-like symptoms. **Stage two** disease (up to 3 months after the tick bite) is accompanied by fever, neck stiffness, headache, lethargy, arthralgias, sore throat, generalized lymphadenopathy, splenomegaly, mononeuritis multiplex (i.e., Bell's palsy), neuropathy, encephalitis, and cardiac complications such as pericarditis and heart block.

Stage three disease occurs months to years later in untreated patients and consists of arthritis and central nervous system manifestations such as memory loss and mood disorders.

Mr. Montgomery has early disseminated Lyme disease (EM with systemic symptoms like headache, malaise, fatigue, and arthralgias). Serologic studies will be ordered, and the patient will be treated with oral antibiotic therapy. Most patients recover without residual deficits. Routine antibiotic prophylaxis for all tick bites is not indicated.

Physical Examination Pearl: Patients who present with Bell's palsy should be screened for Lyme disease. However, the most common cause of bilateral Bell's palsy is Guillain-Barré syndrome.

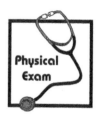

Physical
Exam

Patient Note Pearl: EM is due to the bite of the tick *Ixodes dammini* (the causative agent is *Borrelia burgdorferi*), which causes Lyme disease. In the absence of this rash, Lyme disease may be confused with **other diseases** such as chronic fatigue syndrome or fibromyalgia (these have no joint involvement and tend to be more debilitating). The **diagnostic workup** for Lyme disease should include laboratory confirmation by either indirect immunofluorescence assay (IFA) or the more sensitive and specific enzyme-linked immunosorbent assay (ELISA). A Western blot test is used to confirm the positive ELISA. If the Western blot is negative (for IgM and IgG) in the first 4 weeks of the infection, convalescent titers should be checked, since some patients may be antibody-negative during the early weeks of illness. Patients at high risk for tick bites should be advised to wear long-sleeved shirts and long pants tucked into socks as well as to use insect-repellent sprays.

NOTES

Case 19

The gynecologist in your office building asks you to evaluate Ms. Kandi Kane, 20-year-old college student with hematochezia. Rectal examination performed by the nurse practitioner reveals brown stool with bright red blood and mucus; there are no masses or hemorrhoids.

Vital Signs:

Temperature	98.2°F
Blood pressure	120/75 mmHg
Heart rate	80 beats per minute
Respiratory rate	12 breaths per minute

Examinee's Tasks
(Do not repeat rectal examination)

1. Obtain a focused and relevant history.
2. Perform a focused and relevant physical examination.
3. Discuss your initial diagnostic impressions with the patient.
4. Discuss follow-up tests with the patient.
5. After seeing the patient, complete paperwork relevant to the case.

MY CHECKLIST

History of Present Illness. The Examinee:

1. _____
2. _____
3. _____
4. _____
   _____
5. _____
6. _____
7. _____
8. _____
9. _____
10. _____
11. _____
12. _____
13. _____

Physical Examination. The Examinee:

14. _____
15. _____
16. _____
17. _____
18. _____

Communication Skills. The Examinee:

19. _____
    _____
20. _____
21. _____
22. _____
23. _____
24. _____
25. _____

SP CHECKLIST FOR MS. KANE

History of Present Illness. The Examinee:

____ 1. asked about the onset of rectal bleeding ("It started 3 months ago. It comes and goes.")

____ 2. asked about the frequency of the hematochezia ("It happens once a day.")

____ 3. asked about diarrhea ("Yes; I move my bowels five times a day every day.")

____ 4. asked about abdominal pain ("Sometimes crampy pain in my lower abdomen; but if I have a bowel movement the pain goes away.")

____ 5. asked about nausea or vomiting ("No.")

____ 6. asked about fecal urgency ("Yes; I have to run out of class sometimes to use the ladies room.")

____ 7. asked about tenesmus ("I sit on the toilet an hour sometimes; I feel like I need to go.")

____ 8. asked about mucus in stools ("Yes.")

____ 9. asked about fever ("No.")

____10. asked about weight loss ("Maybe 5 or 6 pounds in the last month.")

____11. asked about recent antibiotic use ("None.")

____12. asked about risk factors for infectious etiology for diarrhea, e.g., recent travel, ill contacts ("None.")

____13. asked about a family history of gastrointestinal problems ("None.")

Physical Examination. The Examinee:

____14. looked in my eyes (conjunctiva and sclerae normal).

____15. listened to my abdomen with a stethoscope (normal bowel sounds auscultated).

____16. tapped over my liver area (no hepatomegaly).

____17. pressed gently throughout my abdomen (no abdominal tenderness).

____18. pressed deeply throughout my abdomen (mild left-lower-quadrant tenderness with deep palpation).

Communication Skills. The Examinee:

____19. explained the initial impression (plausible diagnoses include ulcerative colitis, Crohn's disease, infectious diarrhea).

____20. explained the next steps in the workup (blood work, stool examination, sigmoidoscopy, biopsy).

____21. explained that medications were available for this problem.

____22. explained the prognosis (this chronic problem can be stabilized).

____23. asked about family support system ("My parents are always there for me").

____24. offered to help tell my parents ("Great. Thank you very much").

____25. offered continuous support.

If you performed 18 of these 25 tasks, you passed this test station.

You have 10 minutes to complete your patient note.

HISTORY—Include significant positives and negatives from the history of present illness, past medical history, review of systems, and social and family history.

_____
_____
_____
_____
_____
_____
_____
_____
_____
_____
_____

PHYSICAL EXAMINATION—Indicate only the pertinent positive and negative findings related to the patient's chief complaint.

_____
_____
_____
_____
_____
_____
_____
_____
_____
_____
_____

DIFFERENTIAL DIAGNOSIS—In order of likelihood, write no more than five differential diagnoses for this patient's current problems.

1. _____
2. _____
3. _____
4. _____
5. _____

DIAGNOSTIC WORKUP—Immediate plans for no more than 5 diagnostic studies.

1. _____
2. _____
3. _____
4. _____
5. _____

A SATISFACTORY PATIENT NOTE

HISTORY—Include significant positives and negatives from the history of present illness, past medical history, review of systems, and social and family history.

Ms. Kandi Kane is a 20-year-old college student with no past medical history who presents with a 3-month history of hematochezia. The patient has diarrhea consisting of five bowel movements per day but only one of the daily bowel movements is bloody. She has intermittent crampy lower abdominal pain but no nausea or vomiting. Having a bowel movement relieves the abdominal pain. She has mucus in her stools at times and admits to fecal urgency and tenesmus. She denies fever, recent travel, recent antibiotic use, ill contacts, and family history of gastrointestinal problems. She has had a 5- to 6-lb weight loss over the last 3 months.

PHYSICAL EXAMINATION—Indicate only the pertinent positive and negative findings related to the patient's chief complaint.

The patient is a thin young woman who appears anxious and concerned. Afebrile. BP = 120/75 mmHg. HR = 80 beats/min.
Skin: No rashes.
HEENT: Conjunctivae pink. Sclerae nonicteric.
Lungs: Clear to auscultation.
Heart: Normal S_1 and S_2.
Abdomen: Normal BS. Liver size 10 cm MCL. No splenomegaly. Mild LLQ tenderness with deep palpation. No rebound, rigidity, or guarding.

DIFFERENTIAL DIAGNOSIS
In order of likelihood, write no more than five differential diagnoses for this patient's current problems.

1. Crohn's disease
2. ulcerative colitis
3. hemorrhoids
4. infectious diarrhea
5.

DIAGNOSTIC WORKUP
Immediate plans for no more than five diagnostic studies.

1. CBC
2. electrolytes
3. flexible sigmoidoscopy with biopsy
4. stools for ova and parasites
5.

LEARNING OBJECTIVE FOR MS. KANE
APPROACH TO THE PATIENT WITH HEMATOCHEZIA

Ms. Kandi Kane is a premed student who recently developed hematochezia accompanied by crampy abdominal pain. The pain is relieved after she has a bowel movement. She also complains of urgency and tenesmus. Her stool is bloody and contains mucus. Since this problem began, she has lost 5 pounds.

On physical examination, the patient has normal bowel sounds and mild tenderness with deep palpation. The presentation is most consistent with inflammatory bowel disease (IBD). IBD is more prevalent in whites, particularly Ashkenazi Jews. The sexes are equally affected. There is a higher incidence of IBD in patients with a positive family history, but the patient denies having this risk factor. Infectious diarrhea may present with hematochezia and the stools of this patient need to be evaluated for various bacteria, ova, and parasites. Pseudomembranous colitis from *Clostridium difficile* is unlikely in a patient with no history of antibiotic use. Ischemic colitis would be uncommon in a young woman without a predisposing risk factor.

Ms. Kane will need sigmoidoscopy with biopsy for a definitive diagnosis. The sigmoidoscopy will reveal a uniformly friable and ulcerated colonic mucosa. Biopsy will demonstrate the inflammatory reaction consistent with ulcerative colitis.

The patient will receive medication in an attempt to diminish the symptoms and improve her quality of life. The patient must be informed about the possible systemic complications of IBD, including liver, eye, and skin involvement. The higher incidence of colonic carcinoma in patients with IBD requires an honest and frank discussion with the patient. Close follow-up and surveillance are required for any patient with IBD. The physician must offer Ms. Kane partnership, reassurance, and ongoing support.

Patient Note Pearl: The **differential diagnosis** for hematochezia includes ulcerative colitis, Crohn's disease, hemorrhoids, and infectious diarrhea. Patients with pseudomembranous colitis, ischemic colitis, colon polyps, angiodysplasia, diverticulosis, and malignancy may also present with rectal bleeding. The **diagnostic workup** for the patient should include a CBC to evaluate for anemia or infection, electrolyte measurements to check for abnormalities due to diarrhea, and flexible sigmoidoscopy with possible biopsy. Stools for ova, parasites, *C. difficile* toxin titers, and culture may be sent, but an infectious etiology is less likely.

Case 20

A 41-year-old executive presents to your office with a chief complaint of blurred vision. He went to the optometrist in the shopping mall, who found nothing wrong with his eyesight. The optometrist suggested a checkup from a primary care physician. The patient has not seen a doctor in over 10 years.

The nurse in your practice tells you that the fasting fingerstick glucose level for Mr. David Dunn was 220 mg/dL. Upon entering the examination room, you see an overweight man in no acute distress. His weight is approximately 190 pounds, and he is 5 feet 8 inches tall.

Vital Signs:

Temperature   98.6°F
Blood pressure   130/80 mmHg
Heart rate   86 beats per minute
Respiratory rate   12 breaths per minute

Examinee's Tasks

1. Obtain a focused and relevant history.
2. Perform a focused and relevant physical examination.
3. Discuss your initial diagnostic impressions with the patient.
4. Discuss follow-up tests with the patient.
5. After seeing the patient, complete paperwork relevant to the case.

MY CHECKLIST

History of Present Illness. The Examinee:

1. _____
2. _____
3. _____
4. _____
5. _____
6. _____
7. _____
8. _____
9. _____
10. _____
11. _____
12. _____
13. _____
14. _____

Physical Examination. The Examinee:

15. _____
16. _____
17. _____
18. _____
19. _____
20. _____
21. _____
22. _____
23. _____
24. _____

Communication Skills. The Examinee:

25. _____
26. _____
27. _____
28. _____
29. _____
30. _____
31. _____
32. _____
33. _____

SP CHECKLIST FOR MR. DUNN

History of Present Illness. The Examinee:

___ 1.   asked about the onset of the blurred vision ("It started maybe 2 months ago.")

___ 2.   asked about excessive thirst ("Yes; I have been drinking lots of water lately.")

___ 3.   asked about excessive urination ("Yes; I seem to pass a great amount of urine.")

___ 4.   asked about urgency, hesitancy, or dysuria ("None of that.")

___ 5.   asked about having to go to urinate in the middle of the night ("Yes, every night, at least twice.")

___ 6.   asked about my appetite ("I eat like a horse.")

___ 7.   asked about weight loss ("I have lost about 10 pounds in the last several months and I'm eating more than ever.")

___ 8.   asked about autonomic problems, i.e., impotence, incontinence, dizziness on standing, early satiety from gastroparesis ("I am having problems recently regarding impotence.")

___ 9.   asked about claudication, i.e., pain in the back of my leg when walking ("No.")

___10.   asked about numbness and tingling of my feet ("Yes, that happens all the time now.")

___11.   asked about a family history of diabetes ("My mother uses pills for diabetes.")

___12.   asked about tobacco use ("I have smoked a pack per day for 15 years.")

___13.   asked about alcohol use ("None.")

___14.   asked about any medication use ("None.")

Physical Examination. The Examinee:

___15.   tested my blood pressure lying down and standing (no orthostatic changes in blood pressure).

___16.   looked in my eyes with an ophthalmoscope (normal examination).

___17.   listened over my neck for carotid bruits (no bruits audible).

___18.   felt for PMI over heart (5th ICS in MCL).

___19.   listened to my heart in at least three places (normal examination).

___20.   listened to my lungs in at least four places (normal lung auscultation).

___21.   felt my pulses in both feet (strong pulses palpable bilaterally).

___22.   tested sensation in my legs, i.e., sharp or dull or vibration (decreased sensation in a stocking-like distribution bilaterally).

___23.   used the filament test to screen for loss of pressure sensation (SP cannot feel the filament on either plantar surface).

___24.   checked at least 2 of my reflexes (reflexes normal).

Communication Skills. The Examinee:

___25.   discussed the diagnosis with the patient (diabetes mellitus).

___26.   explained that my mother's having diabetes puts me at risk for the disease.

___27.   explained the physical findings to me (peripheral neuropathy).

___28.   discussed the workup with me (blood work including repeat fasting blood sugar, lipid profile and renal function, urinalysis, electrocardiogram).

___29.   explained the importance of a diabetic diet.

___30.   discussed smoking cessation with me.

___31.   explained that I may need medication if diet fails.

___32.   explained that I would need to check feet often, avoid foot trauma, and choose properly fitting shoes.

___33.   told me that I would learn how to check my own sugar with a glucometer.

If you performed 24 of these 33 tasks, you passed this test station.

You have 10 minutes to complete your patient note.

HISTORY—Include significant positives and negatives from the history of present illness, past medical history, review of systems, and social and family history.

_____
_____
_____
_____
_____
_____
_____
_____
_____
_____

PHYSICAL EXAMINATION—Indicate only the pertinent positive and negative findings related to the patient's chief complaint.

_____
_____
_____
_____
_____
_____
_____
_____
_____

DIFFERENTIAL DIAGNOSIS—In order of likelihood, write no more than five differential diagnoses for this patient's current problems.

1. _____
2. _____
3. _____
4. _____
5. _____

DIAGNOSTIC WORKUP—Immediate plans for no more than five diagnostic studies.

1. _____
2. _____
3. _____
4. _____
5. _____

A SATISFACTORY PATIENT NOTE

HISTORY—Include significant positives and negatives from the history of present illness, past medical history, review of systems, and social and family history.

Mr. David Dunn is a 41-year-old executive who presents with a 2-month history of blurred vision. He has had a 10-lb weight loss despite an excellent appetite; he reports polydypsia, polyuria, and polyphagia. He has no urgency, burning on urination, or hesitancy but has nocturia. He denies dizziness on standing, incontinence, and early satiety but has had occasional erectile dysfunction. He has been experiencing numbness and tingling of his feet but denies claudication. His family history is remarkable for his mother having type 2 diabetes. He denies alcohol use but has smoked 1 pack of cigarettes per day for 15 years. Mr. Dunn has not seen a physician for a checkup in 10 years and takes no medications.

PHYSICAL EXAMINATION—Indicate only the pertinent positive and negative findings related to the patient's chief complaint.

Obese male in NAD. Weight = 190 lb. HT = 68 in. BMI = 28.89 kg/m^2. FS = 220 mg/dl.
BP = 130/80 mmHg and HR = 86 beats/min lying.
BP = 135/83 mmHg and HR = 88 beats/min standing.
HEENT: PERLA. EOMI. No JVD. No carotid bruits. Thyroid gland normal. Fundi: No exudates, hemorrhages, or papilledema.
Heart: PMI 5th ICS MCL. Normal S$_1$ and S$_2$.
Extremities: Dorsalis pedis and posterior tibialis pulses 2+.
Neuro: Decreased sensation to touch bilaterally in stocking-like distribution. Decreased plantar pressure sensation bilaterally.

DIFFERENTIAL DIAGNOSIS
In order of likelihood, write no more than five differential diagnoses for this patient's current problems.

1. diabetes mellitus
2. erectile dysfunction
3. peripheral neuropathy
4. obesity
5.

DIAGNOSTIC WORKUP
Immediate plans for no more than five diagnostic studies.

1. fasting blood sugar
2. electrolytes
3. urinalysis
4. lipid profile
5. electrocardiogram

LEARNING OBJECTIVE FOR MR. DUNN
PROVIDE APPROPRIATE COUNSELING TO A NEW DIABETIC PATIENT

Mr. Dunn has been complaining of blurred vision, polyuria, polydipsia, polyphagia, and weight loss. He has recently developed impotence. He has a family history of diabetes and a fasting fingerstick test in your office reveals a glucose level of 220 mg/dL (a fasting blood glucose of >126 on two occasions would meet the diagnostic criteria for diabetes).

Heart and lung examinations are normal; there are no signs of cardiac decompensation. Neurologic evaluation reveals a peripheral neuropathy. He has no carotid bruits or evidence of peripheral vascular disease.

The patient has several complications of diabetes mellitus. He has neuropathy (both peripheral and autonomic) and needs further evaluation for cardiac dysfunction and microalbuminuria (30 to 300 mg albumin in 24 hours).

The patient requires intensive teaching regarding his diabetes. He must learn how to monitor his own glucose level. He must be instructed about proper diet and smoking cessation. The patient must understand that regular foot care and eye examinations are needed to prevent infections and blindness.

Mr. Dunn should be aware that diabetes is a chronic disease requiring ongoing evaluation and treatment to prevent the life-altering complications of the disease, such as renal failure, infections requiring amputation, stroke, blindness, and cardiomyopathy. The patient must be involved in his own management and enter into a partnership with the physician in an effort to enhance his quality of life. The goals of treatment include a hemoglobin A1c of less than 7 percent and a blood glucose level of 80 to 120 mg/dL.

Physical Examination Pearls: Know the screening test for loss of sensation on the plantar surface of the foot. A 10-g nylon filament is used for this test. If the patient cannot feel this filament, there is loss of pressure sensation and the patient is at risk for foot ulcers (the examinee should remove the shoes and socks of every diabetic patient and examine the feet carefully).

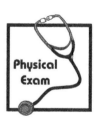

Patient Note Pearl: The **differential diagnosis for blurred vision,** other than diabetes mellitus, includes hypertension, cataracts, macular degeneration, and open-angle glaucoma.

Case 21

A 70-year-old man presents to your office with the chief complaint of difficulty urinating. He is afebrile. Rectal examination performed by the physician assistant is positive for a diffusely enlarged, soft, non-tender prostate gland. No palpable nodules. Stool brown in color. FOBT is negative for blood.

Vital Signs:

Temperature	98.8°F
Blood pressure	123/84 mmHg
Heart rate	85 beats per minute
Respiratory rate	14 breaths per minute

Examinee's Tasks
(Do not repeat the rectal examination)

1. Obtain a focused and relevant history.
2. Perform a focused and relevant physical examination.
3. Discuss your initial diagnostic impressions with the patient.
4. Discuss follow-up tests with the patient.
5. After seeing the patient, complete paperwork relevant to the case.

MY CHECKLIST

History of Present Illness. The Examinee:

1. _____
2. _____
3. _____
4. _____
5. _____
6. _____
   _____
7. _____
8. _____
9. _____
10. _____
11. _____
12. _____
13. _____
14. _____

Physical Examination. The Examinee:

15. _____
16. _____
17. _____

Communication Skills. The Examinee:

18. _____
19. _____
20. _____
21. _____
22. _____
23. _____

SP CHECKLIST FOR MR. LAWTON

History of Present Illness. The Examinee:

___ 1. asked about the onset of difficulty urinating ("It started maybe a month ago.")

___ 2. asked about burning on urination ("No. Not really.")

___ 3. asked about frequency of urination ("I do have to urinate every 3 hours.")

___ 4. asked about nocturia ("I have to get up every night about 3 times.")

___ 5. asked about urgency, i.e., feel like I will not make it to the bathroom on time ("That only happened once.")

___ 6. asked if I felt like I did not completely empty my bladder after urination ("Yes; that's why I think I need to go many times during the day and night; my bladder does not empty.")

___ 7. asked if I needed to strain to urinate ("Yes; I have to push it out sometimes.")

___ 8. asked about any dribbling or a weak stream when urinating ("Yes, that happens sometimes.")

___ 9. asked about hematuria ("No.")

___10. asked about past medical history, i.e., kidney stones, neurologic disease, renal disease ("None.")

___11. asked about weight loss ("No.")

___12. asked about family history of prostate problems, i.e., prostate cancer ("No.")

___13. asked about any medications, i.e., decongestants ("None.")

___14. asked about any fever ("No.")

Physical Examination. The Examinee:

___15. palpated my abdomen (mild suprapubic tenderness).

___16. tapped on my back to elicit costovertebral angle tenderness (no costovertebral angle tenderness).

___17. checked for neurologic deficits in my legs, i.e., sensation, strength, reflexes (normal neurologic exam).

Communication Skills. The Examinee:

___18. explained the results of the physical examination.

___19. explained that my urinary problems may be due to an enlarged prostate.

___20. explained the workup needed (rectal examination, bloodwork for renal function and urinalysis).

___21. explained that medications exist that may help my problem.

___22. established good rapport with me.

___23. was sensitive to my embarrassment.

If you performed 17 of these 23 tasks, you passed this test station.

You have 10 minutes to complete your patient note.

HISTORY—Include significant positives and negatives from the history of present illness, past medical history, review of systems, and social and family history.

_____

_____

_____

_____

_____

_____

_____

_____

_____

_____

PHYSICAL EXAMINATION—Indicate only the pertinent positive and negative findings related to the patient's chief complaint.

_____

_____

_____

_____

_____

_____

_____

_____

_____

DIFFERENTIAL DIAGNOSIS—In order of likelihood, write no more than five differential diagnoses for this patient's current problems.

1. _____

2. _____

3. _____

4. _____

5. _____

DIAGNOSTIC WORKUP—Immediate plans for no more than five diagnostic studies.

1. _____

2. _____

3. _____

4. _____

5. _____

A SATISFACTORY PATIENT NOTE

HISTORY—Include significant positives and negatives from the history of present illness, past medical history, review of systems, and social and family history.

Mr. Linus Lawton is a 70-year-old man with a 1-month history of problems with urination. He denies burning on urination but has frequency and nocturia. After urination, he feels that he has not completely emptied his bladder. He states he experienced one episode of urgency and did not make it the bathroom in time. He often has to strain to urinate and has a weak stream and dribbling when urinating. He denies fever and hematuria. He has no past medical history of kidney stones, renal disease, or neurologic disease. He takes no medications. He has no weight loss or family history of prostate cancer.

PHYSICAL EXAMINATION—Indicate only the pertinent positive and negative findings related to the patient's chief complaint.

Well-developed, well-nourished male in NAD.
Afebrile: BP = 123/84 mmHg. HR = 85 beats/min.
Abdomen: +BS. Positive mild suprapubic tenderness. No rebound. No CVA tenderness.
Rectal: Diffusely enlarged nontender prostate. No nodules. FOBT negative.
Neuro: Sensation to touch normal. Strength 5/5 diffusely. DTR 2+.

DIFFERENTIAL DIAGNOSIS
In order of likelihood, write no more than five differential diagnoses for this patient's current problems.

1. benign prostatic hyperplasia
2. prostate cancer
3. stricture
4. stones
5. neurologic disease

DIAGNOSTIC WORKUP
Immediate plans for no more than five diagnostic studies.

1. urinalysis
2. BUN and creatinine
3. urine culture
4. PSA level measurement
5.

LEARNING OBJECTIVE FOR MR. LAWTON
APPROPRIATELY ASSESS URINARY COMPLAINTS IN THE ELDERLY MALE PATIENT

Mr. Linus Lawton presents with the urinary complaints of frequency, nocturia, urgency, and dribbling. He denies having hematuria. The differential diagnosis for these complaints includes infection, neurologic disease, outlet obstruction from benign prostatic hypertrophy, stricture, stones, and malignancy.

On examination, the patient is found to have suprapubic tenderness and uniform enlargement of the prostate. There is no costovertebral angle tenderness and the patient is afebrile, making infection unlikely. The neurologic examination is normal.

The workup for this patient includes an evaluation of his renal function, since obstruction may cause hydronephrosis and renal impairment. A prostate-specific antigen (PSA) test may be ordered, but a great deal of overlap in levels exists between benign and malignant conditions. Urinalysis will be performed to exclude any infection or hematuria.

The patient may benefit from a 6-month trial of an α-adrenergic blocking agent that inhibits prostatic smooth muscle contraction. Finasteride is another medication used for benign prostatic hypertrophy; it lowers prostatic dihydrotestosterone levels and reduces the size of the prostate. If medical therapy fails, the patient requires urologic evaluation for possible balloon dilatation or surgery. Indications for immediate surgery include renal dysfunction, recurrent stones, hematuria, and persistent urinary retention.

Mr. Lawton should be told to avoid medications such as decongestants that may worsen the obstruction.

Patient Note Pearl: The **differential diagnosis** for this patient includes infection, benign prostatic hypertrophy, neurologic disease, malignancy, stricture, and stones. The **diagnostic workup** includes a CBC to look for infection, electrolyte measurements to evaluate his renal function, urinalysis, and possibly a PSA level measurement.

Case 22

You are the consulting physician for the senior citizens community center and are asked by the social worker to evaluate Mrs. Mildred MacDonald, who is 63 years old. The social worker feels that Mrs. MacDonald has become withdrawn and quiet. In the past, Mrs. MacDonald was extremely sociable and extroverted.

The other senior citizens at the center have noticed the difference and are concerned about the change in their friend as well.

Vital Signs:

Temperature	98.8°F
Blood pressure	130/85 mmHg
Heart rate	88 beats per minute
Respiratory rate	14 breaths per minute

Examinee's Tasks

1. Obtain a focused and relevant history.

2. Assess patient for level of depression and suicide risk.

3. Discuss your initial diagnostic impressions with the patient.

4. Discuss follow-up tests with the patient.

5. After seeing the patient, complete paperwork relevant to the case.

MY CHECKLIST

History of Present Illness. The Examinee:

1. _____
_____

2. _____

3. _____

4. _____

5. _____
_____

6. _____
_____

7. _____

8. _____

9. _____
_____

10. _____
_____

11. _____
_____

12. _____
_____

13. _____
_____

14. _____

15. _____

16. _____
_____

17. _____

Communication Skills. The Examinee:

18. _____

19. _____

20. _____

21. _____

22. _____
_____

23. _____

SP CHECKLIST FOR MRS. MACDONALD

History of Present Illness. The Examinee:

___ 1. asked why I stopped participating in activities ("I don't have the energy anymore; I'm tired of those people in the center; I would rather stay in bed.")

___ 2. asked how long I've had a lack of energy ("Oh, I don't know; for a while now, I guess.")

___ 3. asked about weight loss ("Oh, I'm the same weight as always I guess; I really don't know.")

___ 4. asked about loss of appetite ("Yes; I guess so; I really don't know; I don't feel much like cooking or eating.")

___ 5. asked about difficulty sleeping ("I toss and turn all night trying to sleep; when I do fall asleep, I wake up at 4 A.M.; I'm in bed all day; I sleep all day. If I could, I would be in bed right now.")

___ 6. asked about difficulty concentrating ("I can't even concentrate on reading a newspaper or watching a television show.")

___ 7. asked if I was feeling sad ("Well, I've been happier. I guess I'm sad.")

___ 8. asked if I felt like I was worthless ("Oh, I don't know; I guess I am worthless.")

___ 9. asked if I had feelings of hopelessness ("I am a hopeless case. I guess that would be a good way of putting it.") (SP becomes very tearful at this time.)

___10. asked if anything recently brought on these feelings of sadness ("My husband of 35 years walked out on me 2 months ago; he fell in love with another woman; he has filed for divorce.")

___11. asked if I felt guilty or ashamed about the divorce ("I should have been a better wife, I suppose. I guess it was all my fault. I should have been a better wife. I don't want anyone to know.")

___12. asked about any other support system, like children ("I don't have any family really; we don't have any children; we had a son who drowned when he was 3 years old, but that was a very long time ago.")

___13. asked about a previous history of mood disorder, i.e., psychiatric history ("I needed to be hospitalized for a week or so when my baby drowned, but that was 32 years ago.")

___14. asked about any alcohol use ("None.")

___15. asked about any thoughts of suicide ("Oh, I don't know; I just don't know. The future doesn't look too bright.")

___16. asked about previous attempts at suicide ("Well, when my baby drowned, I did take some pills, but I don't think I really meant to kill myself at that time.")

___17. asked if I had a plan for suicide now ("Oh, I don't know. Well, I do have an old bottle of sleeping pills.")

Communication Skills. The Examinee:

___18. discussed the initial impression with me (plausible diagnosis is depression).

___19. discussed the plan with me (blood work, hospitalization, medications).

___20. was able to draw out the information from me effectively.

___21. responded to my nonverbal clues (tearfulness).

___22. inquired about my feelings regarding the hospitalization ("I really don't care anymore. Do whatever you want, Doctor").

___23. did not become impatient or frustrated with my paucity of speech.

If you performed 17 of these 23 tasks, you passed this test station.

You have 10 minutes to complete your patient note.

HISTORY—Include significant positives and negatives from the history of present illness, past medical history, review of systems, and social and family history.

_____
_____
_____
_____
_____
_____
_____
_____
_____
_____

DIFFERENTIAL DIAGNOSIS—In order of likelihood, write no more than five differential diagnoses for this patient's current problems.

1. _____
2. _____
3. _____
4. _____
5. _____

DIAGNOSTIC WORKUP—Immediate plans for no more than five diagnostic studies.

1. _____
2. _____
3. _____
4. _____
5. _____

A SATISFACTORY PATIENT NOTE

HISTORY—Include significant positives and negatives from the history of present illness, past medical history, review of systems, and social and family history.

Mrs. Mildred MacDonald is a 63-year-old woman who was referred by the social worker at the senior citizen community center for possible depression. In the past, Mrs. MacDonald had been very sociable and extroverted, but she is now withdrawn and quiet. On questioning, Mrs. MacDonald states that she is tired of the people at the community center and prefers to stay in bed. She has difficulty sleeping at night ("tosses and turns"), but when she finally does fall asleep, she wakes up very early in the morning. She feels as if she doesn't have the energy to do things anymore. She has a decrease in appetite but is unsure if she has lost any weight. She does not feel like cooking or eating. She has difficulty concentrating and has stopped reading the newspaper and watching television. She often feels sad, hopeless, and worthless. Her social history is significant for her husband of 35 years leaving her for another woman and filing for divorce. Mrs. MacDonald blames herself for the divorce and feels she should have been a better wife. She has no children; a 3-year-old son died by drowning 32 years ago. Mrs. MacDonald recalls a hospitalization at that time for psychiatric reasons and for taking pills but feels it was not a suicide attempt. She is evasive when questioned about present thoughts of suicide but states she has a bottle of pills at home. She has little hope for the future. The patient is cooperative but is often irritable and indifferent when responding to questions. She is tearful with paucity of speech. If patient is talking about sensitive issues, she does not have good eye contact and her voice is low. Overall, her affect is blunted and her movements are slow. She does not abuse alcohol.

DIFFERENTIAL DIAGNOSIS
In order of likelihood, write no more than 5 differential diagnoses for this patient's current problems.

1. major depressive episode
2. high risk for suicide
3. dysthymic disorder
4. adjustment disorder with depressed mood
5.

DIAGNOSTIC WORKUP
Immediate plans for no more than five diagnostic studies.

1. suicide precautions
2. TSH
3. electrolytes
4. old medical records
5.

LEARNING OBJECTIVE FOR MRS. MACDONALD
SCREEN FOR DEPRESSION AND SUICIDAL IDEATION

Mrs. MacDonald had a previous psychiatric hospital admission following a suicide attempt and depression after the drowning death of her infant son over 30 years ago. Now the patient is expressing feelings of sadness, worthlessness, and hopelessness since her husband of 35 years left her for another woman and filed for divorce. She exhibits psychomotor retardation and has a blunt affect.

Mrs. MacDonald feels a great deal of shame and guilt about the divorce and feels somewhat responsible for her husband's actions. Feelings of shame and guilt often accompany depression.

The patient is fatigued and stays in bed most of the day. She has withdrawn from activities with her friends at the community center. She is anorexic and lacks the concentration to watch a television show or read a newspaper. When she responds to questions, she is irritable and indifferent. The astute physician will realize that Mrs. MacDonald is most likely experiencing a major depressive episode.

The patient with depression may present to the physician's office with a vague complaint such as headache or with severe vegetative signs. Anxiety is present in most depressive disorders. It is not uncommon to observe psychomotor agitation or retardation. The past psychiatric history may reveal a depressive episode.

The physician must screen every depressed patient for suicidal ideation by inquiring about thoughts and plans for suicide. Alcohol use, drug use, male gender, older age, a complete lack of interest in life, or a previous history of a suicide attempt are a few of the factors that make a patient a high risk for suicide. Although Mrs. MacDonald does not drink alcohol, she has several other identifiable factors for suicide and should be hospitalized for inpatient management of her depression. She will benefit from antidepressant medications and psychotherapy. A thorough discussion regarding the side effects of medication use and the length of treatment should take place before Mrs. MacDonald is discharged from the hospital.

History-Taking Pearl: An easy mnemonic used to screen for depression is **SIG E CAPS:**

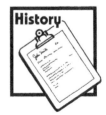

S = **S**leep problems (wakes early and difficulty falling asleep)
I = **I**nterest in life
G = **G**uilt feelings
E = **E**nergy level
C = **C**oncentration
A = **A**ppetite
P = **P**sychomotor retardation or agitation, and
S = **S**uicide (ask about method and suicide note).

Patient Note Pearl: The psychiatric **differential diagnosis** for this patient includes major depression, suicide risk, dysthymic disorder, and adjustment disorder with depressed mood. Medical problems should be excluded by ordering electrolytes and a TSH level. The **workup** may include suicide precautions, support groups, psychotherapy, counseling and use of antidepressants.

NOTES

Case 23

Mr. Jenkins, 40 years old, presents to the emergency room complaining of abdominal pain.

Vital Signs:

Temperature	102.5°F
Blood pressure	130/80 mmHg
Heart rate	110 beats per minute
Respiratory rate	23 breaths per minute

A rectal examination revealed no masses and was FOBT negative. Upon entering the examination room, you see a well-developed man in a hospital gown lying still in the fetal position.

Examinee's Tasks
(Do not repeat rectal examination)

1. Obtain a focused and relevant history.
2. Perform a focused and relevant physical examination.
3. Discuss your initial diagnostic impressions with the patient.
4. Discuss follow-up tests with the patient.
5. After seeing the patient, complete paperwork relevant to the case.

MY CHECKLIST

History of Present Illness. The Examinee:

1. _____
2. _____
3. _____
4. _____
5. _____
6. _____
7. _____
8. _____
9. _____
10. _____
    _____
11. _____
12. _____
13. _____
14. _____
15. _____
16. _____

Physical Examination. The Examinee:

17. _____
18. _____
19. _____
20. _____
21. _____
22. _____
23. _____
    _____

Communication Skills. The Examinee:

24. _____
25. _____
26. _____
27. _____
    _____
28. _____
29. _____
    _____
30. _____

SP CHECKLIST FOR MR. JENKINS

History of Present Illness. The Examinee:

___ 1. asked about the onset of symptoms ("This has been going on nonstop for 2 days.")

___ 2. asked about the location of my pain ("It hurts in the middle of my abdomen.")

___ 3. asked about the quality of my pain ("It's sharp, like a knife going through me.")

___ 4. asked about the radiation of the pain ("It goes all the way through to my back.")

___ 5. asked about the severity of the pain ("On a scale of 1 to 10, where 10 is the worst, it is a 10.")

___ 6. asked about any association with nausea or vomiting ("I cannot stop vomiting.")

___ 7. asked about blood in the vomit ("No.")

___ 8. asked about jaundice ("No.")

___ 9. asked about change in urine color ("No, it's always been yellow.")

___10. asked about a change in bowel movements ("No diarrhea or constipation. My last bowel movement was last night and it was brown.")

___11. asked about any blood in my stools, i.e., tarry stools or bright red blood ("None.")

___12. asked about any alleviating factors ("Lying on my side helps a little.")

___13. asked about any aggravating factors ("Anything I try to eat or drink will worsen the pain; lying flat makes pain worse.")

___14. asked about alcohol use ("Yes, I drink 10 beers every day.")

___15. asked about previous medical problems ("I had an attack of pancreatitis from drinking 2 years ago.")

___16 asked about any medication use ("None.")

Physical Examination. The Examinee:

___17. checked my blood pressure lying down and legs dangling or standing (BP orthostatic changes are present).

___18. checks my eyes (normal conjunctivae and sclerae.)

___19. asked about the onset of periumbilical ecchymosis, i.e., Cullen's sign ("I woke up with it this morning.")

___20. listened with a stethoscope over my abdomen.

___21. palpated gently throughout my abdomen (SP will complain of mild epigastric pain).

___22. palpated deeply throughout the abdomen (SP will complain of severe epigastric pain).

___23. elicited rebound tenderness by pressing my abdomen and then letting go (SP will complain of severe rebound tenderness).

Communication Skills. The Examinee:

___24. seemed to care about my discomfort and pain.

___25. was gentle in eliciting rebound tenderness and during palpation of my abdomen.

___26. explained the physical findings to me.

___27. explained the diagnostic possibilities to me (necrotizing pancreatitis, complicated pancreatitis, peptic ulcer disease, cholelithiasis).

___28. explained that alcohol use was a risk factor for pancreatic disease.

___29. explained the workup for the problem (admission to hospital, intravenous fluids, blood work, radiographic studies, surgical consultation).

___30. explained prognosis (this is a serious condition).

If you performed 21 of these 30 tasks, you passed this test station.

You have 10 minutes to complete your patient note.

HISTORY—Include significant positives and negatives from the history of present illness, past medical history, review of systems, and social and family history.

_____

_____

_____

_____

_____

_____

_____

_____

_____

_____

_____

PHYSICAL EXAMINATION—Indicate only the pertinent positive and negative findings related to the patient's chief complaint.

_____

_____

_____

_____

_____

_____

_____

_____

_____

_____

_____

DIFFERENTIAL DIAGNOSIS—In order of likelihood, write no more than five differential diagnoses for this patient's current problems.

1. _____

2. _____

3. _____

4. _____

5. _____

DIAGNOSTIC WORKUP—Immediate plans for no more than five diagnostic studies.

1. _____

2. _____

3. _____

4. _____

5. _____

A SATISFACTORY PATIENT NOTE

HISTORY—Include significant positives and negatives from the history of present illness, past medical history, review of systems, and social and family history.

Mr. Jenkins is a 40-year-old alcoholic with a past history of pancreatitis who presents with a 2-day history of severe epigastric pain. On a scale of 1 to 10, he describes the pain as a 10. The pain is constant, knife-like in sharpness, and radiates to his back. It is associated with nausea and vomiting but no constipation or diarrhea. His last bowel movement was last night and it was normal. He denies hematemesis, melena, or hematochezia. He has no jaundice or change in urine color. The pain is somewhat alleviated by lying in the fetal position and is worsened by food, liquid, or lying flat. He has no other medical problems and takes no medications. He drinks 10 beers every day.

PHYSICAL EXAMINATION—Indicate only the pertinent positive and negative findings related to the patient's chief complaint.

The patient appears older than his stated age of 40 years. He is lying in the fetal position and appears to be in severe distress. He is asking for an emesis basin.

T = 102.5°F. RR = 23 breaths/min. HR = 110 beats/min.

BP = 130/80 mmHg laying down.

BP = 100/70 mmHg sitting with legs dangling.

HEENT: Conjunctivae pink. Sclerae nonicteric.

Lungs: Normal to auscultation.

Heart: Normal S_1 and S_2. No murmurs, rubs, or gallops.

Abdomen: +BS. Positive Cullen's sign. No Turner's sign.

Severe epigastric pain with palpation.

Positive rebound tenderness.

Rectal exam: No masses. Brown stool. FOBT negative.

DIFFERENTIAL DIAGNOSIS

In order of likelihood, write no more than five differential diagnoses for this patient's current problems.

1. acute pancreatitis
2. necrotizing pancreatitis with hemoperitoneum
3. perforated viscus
4. penetrating ulcer
5.

DIAGNOSTIC WORKUP

Immediate plans for no more than five diagnostic studies.

1. CT scan of the abdomen
2. CBC
3. BUN and creatinine
4. amylase and lipase
5. electrolytes

LEARNING OBJECTIVE FOR MR. JENKINS
RECOGNIZE A SERIOUS COMPLICATION OF A COMMON DISEASE

Mr. Jenkins is an alcoholic patient with a past medical history significant for acute pancreatitis. He presents with severe abdominal pain that radiates to his back and is associated with vomiting. His temperature is elevated and he is in severe abdominal distress. He seems to have some relief when lying in the fetal position. The patient is tachypneic and tachycardic.

The differential diagnosis in this patient includes acute pancreatitis, acute cholecystitis, and perforated viscus. Pancreatitis is the most plausible diagnosis, since the patient still drinks alcohol and has a history of a previous episode of pancreatitis causing similar symptoms. Risk factors for pancreatitis other than alcoholism include medication use, trauma, hyperlipidemia, penetrating ulcer, and biliary diseases such as gallstones. These etiologies are less likely but should still be considered in this patient.

When the patient is undraped for the physical examination, periumbilical discoloration (Cullen's sign) can be seen. There is no flank discoloration or Turner's sign. These findings suggest hemoperitoneum. The patient has rebound tenderness and severe epigastric tenderness with palpation. These physical findings, along with the history, are consistent with the diagnosis of necrotizing pancreatitis. The patient will require blood work for hematologic studies, electrolyte abnormalities, amylase, and lipase. These studies will identify other complications of pancreatitis that may exist in this patient, namely, infection, hypocalcemia, acidosis, and renal dysfunction. Chest and abdominal radiographs may identify a pleural effusion, ascites, or free peritoneal air. A CT scan may be ordered to evaluate the extent of pancreatic necrosis. Vigorous hydration, antibiotics, and other supportive measures are necessary in this patient. The surgical service should be consulted for possible removal of necrotic tissue. Mr. Jenkins should be informed that he has a life-threatening complication of pancreatitis. He will require a great deal of empathy, support, and reassurance.

Patient Note Pearl: The **differential diagnosis** for this patient includes acute pancreatitis, ulcer disease with posterior perforation, and cholecystitis. The **diagnostic workup** may include CBC, electrolytes, BUN, creatinine, glucose, amylase, lipase, serum calcium level, lactate dehydrogenase (LDH) CXR, KUB, and ultrasound or CT scan of the abdomen.

Case 24

Mr. Jack Miller, a 30-year-old businessman, presents to the emergency room complaining of a rash. He was at a restaurant eating a shrimp salad sandwich when he suddenly became red and itchy.

Vital Signs:

Temperature	100.0°F
Blood pressure	120/80 mmHg
Heart rate	105 beats per minute
Respiratory rate	24 breaths per minute

As you enter the room, you see a patient scratching his neck, arms, and legs.

Examinee's Tasks

1. Obtain a focused and relevant history.
2. Perform a focused and relevant physical examination.
3. Discuss your initial diagnostic impressions with the patient.
4. Discuss follow-up tests with the patient.
5. After seeing the patient, complete paperwork relevant to the case.

MY CHECKLIST

History of Present Illness. The Examinee:

1. _____
2. _____
3. _____
4. _____
5. _____
6. _____
7. _____
8. _____
9. _____

Physical Examination. The Examinee:

10. _____
_____
11. _____
12. _____
13. _____

Communication Skills. The Examinee:

14. _____
15. _____
16. _____
_____
17. _____
18. _____
19. _____
20. _____
21. _____

SP CHECKLIST FOR MR. MILLER

History of Present Illness. The Examinee:

___ 1. asked when the rash started ("It started about 40 minutes ago and I came straight to the emergency room.")
___ 2. asked about any difficulty breathing ("Yes, I am feeling a little short of breath.")
___ 3. asked about any chest pain ("My chest does feel tight.")
___ 4. asked about any abdominal distress, i.e., nausea or vomiting ("I do feel nauseated.")
___ 5. asked about a history of allergies in the past, i.e., food or medications ("Never.")
___ 6. asked specifically about allergy to shellfish in the past ("No. I always ate shellfish without any problems.")
___ 7. asked about a history of asthma ("No.")
___ 8. asked about a family history of allergies ("No.")
___ 9. asked about medications I take, i.e., ACE inhibitors, beta blockers ("No.")

Physical Examination. The Examinee:

___10. asked me to remove my shirt to look at the rash more carefully (SP will have erythematous rash throughout trunk, neck, arms, and legs, with scattered scratch marks).
___11. looked inside my mouth (normal examination).
___12. listened to my lungs in at least four places (audible bilateral inspiratory and expiratory wheezes).
___13. listened to my heart in at least three places (normal examination).

Communication Skills. The Examinee:

___14. explained the diagnosis to me (allergic reaction or anaphylaxis).
___15. explained that the allergy was most likely due to shellfish.
___16. explained the treatment to me (injection of epinephrine, beta-agonist agent via nebulizer, oxygen, antihistamines, H_2 blockers, and steroids).
___17. explained that arrangements would be made for me to be seen by an allergist.
___18. told me that in the future I would need to wear a medical alert bracelet.
___19. told me that in the future I would need to carry a pen with medication to start self-treatment if needed.
___20. conveyed a sense of confidence.
___21. made me feel at ease.

If you performed 16 of these 21 tasks, you passed this test station.

You have 10 minutes to complete your patient note.

HISTORY—Include significant positives and negatives from the history of present illness, past medical history, review of systems, and social and family history.

_____

_____

_____

_____

_____

_____

_____

_____

_____

_____

PHYSICAL EXAMINATION—Indicate only the pertinent positive and negative findings related to the patient's chief complaint.

_____

_____

_____

_____

_____

_____

_____

_____

_____

DIFFERENTIAL DIAGNOSIS—In order of likelihood, write no more than five differential diagnoses for this patient's current problems.

1. _____

2. _____

3. _____

4. _____

5. _____

DIAGNOSTIC WORKUP—Immediate plans for no more than five diagnostic studies.

1. _____

2. _____

3. _____

4. _____

5. _____

A SATISFACTORY PATIENT NOTE

HISTORY—Include significant positives and negatives from the history of present illness, past medical history, review of systems, and social and family history.

Mr. Jack Miller is a 30-year-old businessman who developed a pruritic skin rash while eating a shrimp salad sandwich at a local restaurant. He reports that "the symptoms started 40 minutes ago" and he came straight to the emergency room. He feels very short of breath and has some chest tightness. He feels nauseated but has no vomiting. He has no food or medication allergies and has eaten shrimp in the past without any difficulty. He takes no medications and has no family history of allergies. He has no history of asthma.

PHYSICAL EXAMINATION—Indicate only the pertinent positive and negative findings related to the patient's chief complaint.

The patient is a well-developed, well-nourished male in moderate discomfort. He is scratching his neck, chest, arms, and thighs.
BP = 120/80 mmHg. HR = 105 beats/min. RR = 24 breaths/min.
T = 100.0°F.
Skin: Diffuse erythematous rash is visible over arms, legs, thighs, and chest. No hives are visible. Positive for scratch marks.
HEENT: Throat without erythema. Tongue and uvula normal in size.
Lungs: Scattered mild inspiratory and expiratory wheezes. Good air entry.
Heart: Normal S_1 and S_2. No murmurs.

DIFFERENTIAL DIAGNOSIS
In order of likelihood, write no more than five differential diagnoses for this patient's current problems.

1. allergic reaction
2. angioedema
3. asthma
4.
5.

DIAGNOSTIC WORKUP
Immediate plans for no more than five diagnostic studies.

1. pulse oximetry reading for oxygen saturation
2. CBC for eosinophilia
3. CXR
4. peak flow measurement
5.

LEARNING OBJECTIVE FOR MR. MILLER
EVALUATE THE PATIENT WITH RASH

Mr. Jack Miller has no previous history of allergies or allergic reactions and has eaten shellfish in the past without problem. He presents with pruritus, flushing, chest tightness, nausea, and difficulty breathing after eating a shrimp salad sandwich. On physical examination, his skin is erythematous; his lung findings are significant for bilateral inspiratory and expiratory wheezes. The patient needs treatment with 1:1000 subcutaneous epinephrine, H_1 (diphenhydramine) and H_2 blockers, albuterol, steroids, and oxygen. Anaphylaxis is an IgE (found on mast cells)-mediated reaction. These reactions are most commonly due to medications such as penicillin and cephalosporins, foods, insect bites, and latex. Anaphylaxis presents with chest pain, wheezing, urticaria, or angioedema. The patient may be hypotensive and tachycardic. Angioedema and urticaria are cutaneous forms of anaphylaxis. Angioedema, unlike urticaria, occurs in the deeper subcutaneous tissues. It may be acquired (use of an ACE inhibitor is often a cause) or may be due to an autosomal dominant congenital (C_1 esterase inhibitor) deficiency. Angioedema has been associated with malignant diseases such as lymphoma, leukemia, and adenocarcinoma.

Patient Note Pearl: The **differential diagnosis** includes allergic reaction, asthma, and angioedema. The **workup** may include a pulse oximetry reading, peak flow measurement, and allergy testing.

Case 25

A 31-year-old woman named Wendy Walker presents to your office complaining of right wrist pain. She states that a fall down the stairs caused the injury. She is concerned that the wrist may be fractured.

Vital Signs:

Temperature	99.0°F
Blood pressure	120/80 mmHg
Heart rate	75 beats per minute
Respiratory rate	14 breaths per minute

Upon entering the examination room, you notice a somewhat nervous woman pacing back and forth in the room constantly looking at her watch. She appears older than her stated age.

Examinee's Tasks

1. Obtain a focused and relevant history.
2. Perform a focused and relevant physical examination.
3. Discuss your initial diagnostic impressions with the patient.
4. Discuss follow-up tests with the patient.
5. After seeing the patient, complete paperwork relevant to the case.

MY CHECKLIST

History of Present Illness. The Examinee:

1. _____
2. _____
3. _____
4. _____
5. _____
6. _____
   _____
7. _____
   _____
8. _____
   _____
9. _____
10. _____
    _____
11. _____
12. _____
    _____
13. _____
14. _____
    _____

Physical Examination. The Examinee:

15. _____

Communication Skills. The Examinee:

16. _____
17. _____
18. _____
19. _____
20. _____
21. _____
22. _____
23. _____
24. _____

SP CHECKLIST FOR MRS. WALKER

History of Present Illness. The Examinee:

___ 1. asked how the wrist injury happened ("I fell down a flight of stairs; it was an accident.")

___ 2. asked when the accident happened ("About 1 hour ago.")

___ 3. asked about any other injuries ("Maybe a few bruises, but nothing major.")

___ 4. asked about any other medical problems ("None.")

___ 5. asked about any medication use ("No.")

___ 6. asked about the bruises on my arms (SP has many bruises painted on her arms; some appear old) ("I guess I got them from falling down the flight of stairs today.")

___ 7. asked whether my husband was physically abusive ("He hits me sometimes; that's what happened today; it only happens when he drinks. It's my fault though, since I make him angry sometimes.")

___ 8. asked about my children ("Yes, we have two children, 5 and 7 years old. My 7-year-old son is starting to act a little like my husband already.")

___ 9. asked if my husband ever abused the children ("No. Never.")

___10. asked me if I felt safe at home ("Not really; I never know when my husband is going to become angry with me; he drinks almost every day now.")

___11. asked me if I was afraid at home ("Sometimes.")

___12. asked if any family or close friends knew about the abuse ("He would kill me or take the children away if I told anyone.")

___13. asked me if there were any guns at home ("He has a gun collection; he likes to hunt.")

___14. asked me if I had any emergency plan for where to go if I needed to leave my husband ("I guess I would go to a shelter with the children; I don't know.")

Physical Examination. The Examinee:

___15. checked for full range of motion at the wrist (normal wrist examination except for bruises).

Communication Skills. The Examinee:

___16. informed me that spousal abuse was illegal.

___17. told me that involving the police helps prevent further abuse.

___18. told me that I did not deserve to be abused.

___19. informed me that violence in the home affects the future behavior of children.

___20. acknowledged that leaving an abusive husband is very difficult to do.

___21. showed concern for my safety.

___22. offered ongoing support, guidance, and counseling.

___23. discussed available support groups in the community (emergency telephone numbers and shelters).

___24. discussed safety and exit plans.

If you performed 17 of these 24 tasks, you passed this test station.

You have 10 minutes to complete your patient note.

HISTORY—Include significant positives and negatives from the history of present illness, past medical history, review of systems, and social and family history.

_____
_____
_____
_____
_____
_____
_____
_____
_____
_____
_____

PHYSICAL EXAMINATION—Indicate only the pertinent positive and negative findings related to the patient's chief complaint.

_____
_____
_____
_____
_____
_____
_____
_____
_____
_____
_____

DIFFERENTIAL DIAGNOSIS—In order of likelihood, write no more than five differential diagnoses for this patient's current problems.

1. _____
2. _____
3. _____
4. _____
5. _____

DIAGNOSTIC WORKUP—Immediate plans for no more than five diagnostic studies.

1. _____
2. _____
3. _____
4. _____
5. _____

A SATISFACTORY PATIENT NOTE

HISTORY—Include significant positives and negatives from the history of present illness, past medical history, review of systems, and social and family history.

Wendy Walker is a 31-year-old woman with the chief complaint of right wrist pain. She states that she accidentally fell down the stairs an hour ago and is concerned that her wrist might be fractured. She thinks that she might have a few other bruises as a result of the fall but feels that these are not significant. She has come for a medical evaluation of her right wrist. She has no past medical history and takes no medications. When questioned about other bruises on her arms, some of them old, the patient states that they are from today's fall as well. With further questioning, the patient admits that her husband occasionally hits her, which is what happened today, but states that he is abusive only when he is drinking alcohol. She also feels that she must be doing something wrong to get him angry enough to hit her. She has two children, ages 5 and 7, but states that her husband never abuses them. She feels, however, that her older son is starting to act angry, like his father. At present, she does not feel safe at home, because her husband is drinking daily and it is unpredictable when he will become angry with her. She sometimes feels afraid at home. She has not told family and friends about the abuse because she thinks her husband would kill her or take away the children if she were to tell anyone. Her husband is an avid hunter and there are many guns in the home. Although the patient states that she would go to a women's shelter with the children in case things got out of hand, she really has no emergency plan to leave her husband if that should ever become necessary.

PHYSICAL EXAMINATION—Indicate only the pertinent positive and negative findings related to the patient's chief complaint.

The patient appears older than her stated age of 31 years. She is somewhat nervous and is pacing back and forth in the room. She is constantly looking at her watch to check the time. She is guarded and defensive when responding to questions. VS normal.
Skin: Many ecchymoses on arms; some appear older than 1 day.
Right wrist: 2-cm area of ecchymosis. Full ROM. No pain or tenderness with palpation.

DIFFERENTIAL DIAGNOSIS

In order of likelihood, write no more than five differential diagnoses for this patient's current problems.

1. spousal abuse
2. ecchymosis of right wrist
3. multiple ecchymoses of the upper extremities
4. right wrist sprain
5.

DIAGNOSTIC WORKUP

Immediate plans for no more than five diagnostic studies.

1. safety plan
2. counseling
3. develop support system
4. bandage for right wrist
5.

LEARNING OBJECTIVE FOR MRS. WALKER
IDENTIFY AND HELP THE VICTIM OF DOMESTIC VIOLENCE

The victim of domestic violence is often restless and guarded and checks her watch frequently (husband has her timed). She will be reluctant to give information unless the physician is supportive and nonjudgmental. A patient may present with a poorly explained injury, especially to the face; an obvious laceration, bruise, or fracture; or with a subtle pain-related complaint such as recurrent headache, chest pain, or abdominal pain (irritable bowel). Physicians should routinely screen for domestic violence not only in the emergency room but in the office setting as well (1 in 5 patients who present to a primary care practice are involved in a relationship where abuse exists).

Mrs. Walker presents with a bruise to her wrist and has evidence of older bruises. She explains these injuries poorly by stating that she fell down a flight of stairs. The patient admits that her husband drinks and abuses her physically. The history of her husband's alcoholism is important to obtain, since half of all domestic violence cases are associated with alcohol or drug abuse.

The physician should inquire about the safety of the children and the presence of firearms in the home. Spousal abuse is repetitive and may lead to murder of the spouse and abuse of the children. The victim should be informed that spousal abuse is illegal and that informing the police of the situation may help prevent further abuse.

It is often difficult for women to leave the abuser, and the physician should acknowledge this. Finances (fear of not being able to adequately support the children) and fear of suffering more abuse (escalating abuse) because of leaving are the reasons victims remain in abusive relationships.

The physician should, first, tell the patient that she does not deserve to be abused. The doctor should present the options to Mrs. Walker and offer to contact a support group where women with similar situations will be able to help her. The wife and children may be able to move to a "safe house," where the patient can review her options carefully without the threat of violence. The wife should never be told by the physician to leave the husband immediately. The patient should be allowed to make her own decisions, since this is an important step in the treatment and recovery of the abused patient. The physician should, however, offer continuous support and be available for future guidance and counseling and should help the patient develop a safety plan: a suitcase left with a friend or relative with essential clothing for the patient and children, necessary medications, car keys, driver's license, money, checkbook, social security numbers, savings account book, birth certificates, and special toys or books for the children.

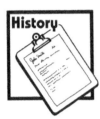

History-Taking Pearl: Remember the **SAFE** questionnaire for domestic violence screening:

S = Do you feel **s**afe or **s**tressed in relationships?
A = Have you ever been **a**bused or **a**fraid in a relationship?
F = Are your **f**riends and **f**amily aware of your relationship problem?
E = Do you have an **e**mergency plan if needed?

NOTES

Case 26

A 50-year-old secretary named Mildred Payne is in your office complaining of tingling in her left hand. She feels this is an early sign of a stroke and requests to be seen immediately. Her usual physician is your partner, who has the day off to testify at a malpractice hearing. The patient has no appointment scheduled but is making such a scene in your waiting room that you decide to see her.

Vital Signs:

Temperature	98.6°F
Blood pressure	130/80 mmHg
Heart rate	76 beats per minute
Respiratory rate	14 breaths per minute

Examinee's Tasks

1. Obtain a focused and relevant history.

2. Perform a focused and relevant physical examination.

3. Discuss your initial diagnostic impressions with the patient.

4. Discuss follow-up tests with the patient.

5. After seeing the patient, complete paperwork relevant to the case.

MY CHECKLIST

History of Present Illness. The Examinee:

1. _____
2. _____
3. _____
4. _____
5. _____
6. _____
7. _____
   _____
8. _____
9. _____
10. _____

Physical Examination. The Examinee:

11. _____
12. _____
13. _____
14. _____
15. _____
    _____
16. _____

Communication Skills. The Examinee:

17. _____
18. _____
19. _____
20. _____
    _____
21. _____
22. _____
23. _____
24. _____

SP CHECKLIST FOR MRS. PAYNE

History of Present Illness. The Examinee:

___ 1. asked about the onset of hand tingling ("It started last night before I went to bed and now it's worse.")

___ 2. asked about weakness of the hand ("I think my thumb is a little weak.")

___ 3. asked about the distribution of the tingling ("It is worse in my middle and index fingers.")

___ 4. asked about radiation of the tingling to the arm or neck ("No.")

___ 5. asked about any aggravating factors ("Sleeping and driving.")

___ 6. asked about any alleviating factors ("Shaking my hand makes it go away a little.")

___ 7. asked about signs of a stroke, i.e., speech difficulty, vision changes, face, arm, or leg numbness or weakness ("No.")

___ 8. asked about repetitive movement at work ("Yes. I've done data entry on a keyboard all day for 10 years.")

___ 9. asked about handedness ("I am left-handed.")

___10. asked about history of diseases, such as rheumatoid arthritis, diabetes, or hypothyroidism ("No illnesses.")

Physical Examination. The Examinee:

___11. tested muscle strength in my upper arm (normal strength).

___12. tested muscle strength in my left lower arm (normal strength).

___13. tested biceps or triceps reflex of my left arm (normal).

___14. tested muscle strength of the fingers in my left hand (thumb flexion is weak).

___15. tested sensation by pinprick in my left hand (decreased sensation over the palmar aspect of left thumb, index, and middle fingers).

___16. tapped over my left wrist (SP will complain of severe tingling of the left hand; positive Tinel's sign).

Communication Skills. The Examinee:

___17. acknowledged my distress.

___18. showed empathy.

___19. did not become impatient or frustrated with me.

___20. discussed the diagnostic possibilities with me (i.e., carpal tunnel syndrome, cervical radiculopathy, ulnar neuropathy).

___21. talked about the plan (electromyography and splinting of the hand).

___22. talked about prognosis (good).

___23. checked my understanding of the problem.

___24. reassured me that I was not having a stroke.

If you performed 17 of these 24 tasks, you passed this test station.

You have 10 minutes to complete your patient note.

HISTORY—Include significant positives and negatives from the history of present illness, past medical history, review of systems, and social and family history.

_____

_____

_____

_____

_____

_____

_____

_____

_____

_____

PHYSICAL EXAMINATION—Indicate only the pertinent positive and negative findings related to the patient's chief complaint.

_____

_____

_____

_____

_____

_____

_____

_____

_____

_____

DIFFERENTIAL DIAGNOSIS—In order of likelihood, write no more than five differential diagnoses for this patient's current problems.

1. _____

2. _____

3. _____

4. _____

5. _____

DIAGNOSTIC WORKUP—Immediate plans for no more than five diagnostic studies.

1. _____

2. _____

3. _____

4. _____

5. _____

A SATISFACTORY PATIENT NOTE

HISTORY—Include significant positives and negatives from the history of present illness, past medical history, review of systems, and social and family history.

Ms. Mildred Payne is a 50-year-old woman who emergently presents complaining of left-hand tingling. She states that the tingling began the night before but has been progressively worsening. She states that the tingling is especially bad in her left middle and index fingers. Additionally, she feels that her thumb is weak. There is no tingling in her arm or neck. The other hand is normal. Sleeping and driving make the tingling worse, but shaking her hand a little alleviates the symptoms. She denies speech difficulty, vision changes, or any other numbness, tingling, and weakness. She is employed as a computer data-entry technician. She denies a history of diabetes mellitus, hypothyroidism, or rheumatoid arthritis.

PHYSICAL EXAMINATION—Indicate only the pertinent positive and negative findings related to the patient's chief complaint.

The patient is a very anxious and worried woman who looks her stated age of 50.
She is concerned that she may be having a stroke.
VS: Normal.
Neuro: Alert and oriented ×3. CN II-XII normal. Left-handed.
Strength: Weak left thumb flexion, otherwise normal.
Sensory: Decreased sensation to dull and sharp over palmar aspect of left 1st, 2nd, and 3rd digits.
Positive Tinel's sign. Positive Phalen's sign.
Rest of sensory examination is normal.
DTR: 2+ diffusely.

DIFFERENTIAL DIAGNOSIS
In order of likelihood, write no more than five differential diagnoses for this patient's current problems.

1. carpal tunnel syndrome
2. cervical radiculopathy
3. ulnar neuropathy
4. thoracic outlet syndrome
5.

DIAGNOSTIC WORKUP
Immediate plans for no more than five diagnostic studies.

1. electromyography
2. splinting of left hand
3.
4.
5.

LEARNING OBJECTIVE FOR MRS. PAYNE
REASSURING THE ANXIOUS PATIENT

Ms. Payne complains of left-hand tingling that is worse when driving and sleeping and improves with hand shaking. She denies having radiation of her symptoms and has no stroke-related complaints. The tingling is confined to her first, second, and third digits. On further questioning, the patient complains of mild weakness of her left thumb. These complaints localize the problem to the median nerve distribution.

Carpal tunnel syndrome occurs when there is compression or entrapment of the median nerve underneath the flexor retinaculum due to injury from overuse, obesity, pregnancy, or systemic diseases such as diabetes mellitus, acromegaly, amyloidosis, hypothyroidism, gout, and rheumatoid arthritis. The repetitive movements performed by Mrs. Payne in her job as a computer data-entry technician may have caused her problem.

On physical examination, Mrs. Payne is found to have normal arm strength and reflexes. There is weakness in flexion of the first digit, and sensory loss, elicited by pinprick, is found in the distribution of the median nerve. When the median nerve at the wrist is tapped, tingling of the hand (Tinel's sign) occurs. Phalen's sign or tingling from wrist flexion could also be positive in carpal tunnel syndrome.

Electromyography is the best method to diagnose carpal tunnel syndrome. Fifty percent of patients who present with unilateral carpal tunnel syndrome actually have bilateral disease. Treatment includes splinting of the hand, anti-inflammatory agents, elevation, and steroid injection directly into the median nerve. Further trauma or injury to the hand should be avoided. The patient requires reassurance that the symptoms she is experiencing are unrelated to a stroke.

Physical Examination Pearl: Normal limb compartment tissue pressure is 8 mmHg. In carpal tunnel syndrome, the pressure may be 30 mmHg at rest and may go as high as 90 mmHg with flexion (Phalen's sign is a more sensitive sign than Tinel's sign).

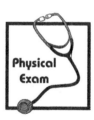

Patient Note Pearl: The **differential diagnosis** for this patient's presentation includes carpal tunnel syndrome, transient ischemic attack, cervical radiculopathy (pain would radiate proximally to the shoulder), ulnar neuropathy (fifth digit and medial hand numbness), and thoracic outlet syndrome (sensory loss over the ulnar side of the hand and forearm and weakness of all the hand muscles). The "gold standard" for diagnosis of carpal tunnel syndrome is electromyography.

Case 27

Daniel Doolittle is a 33-year-old salesman who makes an appointment to see you because of a backache. He is asking your office manager to schedule him for a magnetic resonance imaging (MRI) study to evaluate his back problem. Mr. Doolittle states that his friend had a similar backache and he needed an MRI, so why not just order one for him too?

Mr. Doolittle had his annual physical examination 3 months ago, and it was normal. He has no medical problems and takes no medications.

Vital Signs:

Temperature	98.6°F
Blood pressure	120/80 mmHg
Heart rate	86 beats per minute
Respiratory rate	12 breaths per minute

Examinee's Tasks

1. Obtain a focused and relevant history.
2. Perform a focused and relevant physical examination.
3. Discuss your initial diagnostic impressions with the patient.
4. Discuss follow-up tests with the patient.
5. After seeing the patient, complete paperwork relevant to the case.

MY CHECKLIST

History of Present Illness. The Examinee:

1. _____
_____
2. _____
3. _____
4. _____
5. _____
_____
6. _____
7. _____
8. _____
9. _____
10. _____
11. _____

Physical Examination. The Examinee:

12. _____
13. _____
14. _____
15. _____
16. _____
17. _____
18. _____
19. _____
20. _____

Communication Skills. The Examinee:

21. _____
22. _____
23. _____
24. _____
25. _____
26. _____

CHECKLIST FOR MR. DOOLITTLE

History of Present Illness. The Examinee:

___ 1. asked about the location of my back pain ("It is in the middle of my lower back.") (SP points to L4 and L5 vertebral body areas.)

___ 2. asked about the onset of my back pain ("It started yesterday. Took 2 Tylenol and it didn't help.")

___ 3. asked about the quality of my pain ("It is like a dull, throbbing pain.")

___ 4. asked about the frequency of the pain ("It is continuous.")

___ 5. asked about any alleviating factors ("Lying still on my back in bed or lying on one side with my knees bent helps a little.")

___ 6. asked about any aggravating factors ("Bending, standing, walking, sitting, coughing, and sneezing make it worse.")

___ 7. asked about any precipitating event ("It started when I moved my computer monitor to my new office.")

___ 8. asked about any leg weakness ("No.")

___ 9. asked about any sensory changes in my back or legs ("No.")

___10. asked about any bowel and bladder incontinence ("None.")

___11. asked about any history of back problems in the past ("No.")

Physical Examination. The Examinee:

___12. tested for back tenderness with fingers (tender lower back).

___13. tested muscle strength in both of my legs (normal strength).

___14. tested sensation in both of my legs (normal sensation).

___15. tested reflexes in both of my legs (normal reflexes).

___16. checked my plantar or Babinski reflex by scratching the soles of my feet (toes are downgoing bilaterally).

___17. performed straight leg raising in both legs (no pain with straight leg raising).

___18. evaluated my spine for range of motion in all directions (SP complains of some pain when bending forward).

___19. assessed my gait by asking me to walk (normal gait).

___20. asked me to walk on toes or heels (normal).

Communication Skills. The Examinee:

___21. acknowledged my discomfort.

___22. discussed the problem with me (most likely back sprain; herniated disk and sciatica less likely).

___23. discussed treatment (bed rest for 3 days, mobilization as tolerated, nonsteroidal anti-inflammatory drugs).

___24. gave clear reasons why the MRI was not needed.

___25. did not belittle or ignore my request for an MRI.

___26. scheduled a follow-up appointment to see me.

If you performed 19 of these 26 tasks, you passed this test station.

You have 10 minutes to complete your patient note.

HISTORY—Include significant positives and negatives from the history of present illness, past medical history, review of systems, and social and family history.

_____

_____

_____

_____

_____

_____

_____

_____

_____

_____

PHYSICAL EXAMINATION—Indicate only the pertinent positive and negative findings related to the patient's chief complaint.

_____

_____

_____

_____

_____

_____

_____

_____

_____

_____

DIFFERENTIAL DIAGNOSIS—In order of likelihood, write no more than five differential diagnoses for this patient's current problems.

1. _____

2. _____

3. _____

4. _____

5. _____

DIAGNOSTIC WORKUP—Immediate plans for no more than five diagnostic studies.

1. _____

2. _____

3. _____

4. _____

5. _____

A SATISFACTORY PATIENT NOTE

HISTORY—Include significant positives and negatives from the history of present illness, past medical history, review of systems, and social and family history.

Mr. Daniel Doolittle is a 33-year-old salesman who complains of having had lower back pain for 1 day. The pain is throbbing and dull in nature and is continuous. The pain is aggravated by bending, standing, walking, sitting, coughing, and sneezing and is alleviated by lying flat on his back or on his side with his knees bent. He had no relief with 2 Tylenol tablets. The pain began at work after the patient lifted and moved his computer monitor from one office to another. There is no radiation of the pain down his legs and he denies weakness, numbness, and tingling of his legs. He has no bladder or bowel incontinence. He has never had back problems in the past. He has no past medical history and his annual checkup 3 months ago was normal.

PHYSICAL EXAMINATION—Indicate only the pertinent positive and negative findings related to the patient's chief complaint.

The patient is a well-developed, well-nourished male. He is asking for an emergency MRI to evaluate his back problem. He is grimacing due to pain and is impatient with questions.
VS normal.
Neuro: Motor: Strength 5/5 LE bilaterally.
Sensory: Sensation intact to touch and pinprick.
Bilaterally LE Reflexes: 2+ knee and ankle jerk.
Babinski: Negative.
Musculoskeletal: Back with full ROM.
Point tenderness over L4 and L5.
Negative straight leg raise maneuver bilaterally.
Gait: Normal. Able to walk on heels and toes without difficulty.

DIFFERENTIAL DIAGNOSIS
In order of likelihood, write no more than five differential diagnoses for this patient's current problems.

1. back strain
2. herniated disk
3. sciatic nerve irritation
4. arthritis
5.

DIAGNOSTIC WORKUP
Immediate plans for no more than five diagnostic studies.

1. bed rest
2. out of bed as tolerated
3. rectal examination to check rectal tone
4. pain relief
5.

LEARNING OBJECTIVE FOR MR. DOOLITTLE
EVALUATE BACK PAIN

The differential diagnosis for back pain includes sprain, arthritis, spinal stenosis, herniated disk, tumor, infection such as osteomyelitis, sciatic nerve irritation, and ankylosing spondylitis. Mr. Doolittle complains of low back pain that occurred after lifting a heavy computer monitor. The pain does not radiate to the lower extremities and is not accompanied by neurologic symptoms such as incontinence or sensory deficit. Bladder and bowel dysfunction (cauda equina syndrome) and sensory abnormalities may be seen with disk herniation.

The pain experienced by Mr. Doolittle does not improve with activity. The back pain of ankylosing spondylitis usually lessens as activity increases. Mr. Doolittle had a normal physical examination 3 months ago, which makes tumor and chronic infection less likely. Disk pain worsens with coughing, bending, and sitting but improves with standing (decreases disk pressure). Mr. Doolittle's back pain worsens with standing.

The physical examination performed on Mr. Doolittle reveals no sensory or motor deficits, and his reflexes are normal. His gait is assessed as normal, and he has minimal lumbar pain with forward flexion of the spine. He has point tenderness with palpation of L4 and L5.

Straight leg raising often helps to differentiate between sciatic nerve irritation, where symptoms of back pain worsen with elevation of the involved extremity, and disk herniation, where pain is elicited with minimal leg elevation bilaterally. Herniation may also produce a positive "crossed" straight leg raising test. Mr. Doolittle has no worsened symptoms with straight leg raising. The most likely diagnosis in this patient is back sprain, and the optimal treatment would be minimal bed rest with mobilization as tolerated. Nonsteroidal anti-inflammatory drugs for pain relief should be prescribed. The physician must explain the diagnosis to Mr. Doolittle and reassure him that radiographic studies, including MRI, are not appropriate at this time.

History-Taking Pearl: Pseudoclaudication with low back pain may indicate spinal stenosis. The back pain of spinal stenosis is relieved by leaning forward (flexion) and by squatting.

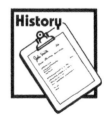

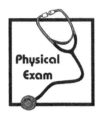

Physical Examination Pearl: Palpation of the spine for point tenderness is not a good diagnostic test, and it yields little information. Point tenderness, if present, may indicate osteomyelitis.

The Schober test helps diagnose ankylosing spondylitis. A measuring tape is placed 10 cm above and 5 cm below the S$_1$ area. The patient is asked to flex as far down as possible. The tape should distract 5 cm or more for normal lumbar motion.

Patient Note Pearl: The **differential diagnosis** for this patient includes back sprain, sciatic nerve irritation, arthritis, and herniated disk. The **diagnostic workup** may include a rectal examination to check for sphincter tone, bed rest, the initiation of nonsteroidal anti-inflammatory drugs, and mobilization as tolerated.

NOTES

Case 28

A 17-year-old high school senior named Jane Jett is brought to the emergency room by the school nurse because of shortness of breath.

Vital Signs:

Temperature	98.6°F
Blood pressure	100/70 mmHg
Respiratory rate	28 breaths per minute
Heart rate	100 beats per minute
Oxygen saturation	99%

Upon entering the examination room, you observe an adolescent who is in mild respiratory distress. She seems to be frightened and concerned. She is looking at the peak flowmeter and appears to be perplexed.

Examinee's Tasks

1. Obtain a focused and relevant history.
2. Perform a focused and relevant physical examination.
3. Discuss your initial diagnostic impressions with the patient.
4. Discuss follow-up tests with the patient.
5. After seeing the patient, complete paperwork relevant to the case.

MY CHECKLIST

History of Present Illness. The Examinee:

1. _____
2. _____
3. _____
   _____
   _____
4. _____
5. _____
6. _____
7. _____
8. _____
9. _____
10. _____
11. _____
12. _____
13. _____

Physical Examination. The Examinee:

14. _____
15. _____

Communication Skills. The Examinee:

16. _____
17. _____
18. _____
19. _____
20. _____
21. _____
22. _____
23. _____
24. _____
25. _____
26. _____

SP CHECKLIST FOR JANE JETT

History of Present Illness. The Examinee:

___ 1. asked about the onset of the shortness of breath ("It started 2 hours ago.")

___ 2. asked what I was doing at the time the shortness of breath started ("Running in gym class.")

___ 3. asked about problems with shortness of breath and exercise before ("Something like this happened last month while I was playing basketball during gym class and last week while I was running to get to class, but the breathing always returns to normal in an hour.")

___ 4. asked about chest tightness ("I do feel like my chest is a little tight.")

___ 5. asked about cough ("No.")

___ 6. asked about any recent upper respiratory tract infections ("None.")

___ 7. asked about past medical history ("I've never been sick before.")

___ 8. asked about any medications ("Just vitamins.")

___ 9. asked about any history of allergies ("None.")

___10. asked about a history of rashes ("No.")

___11. asked about a family history of asthma ("No.")

___12. asked about smoking ("No.")

___13. asked about illicit drug use ("None.")

Physical Examination. The Examinee:

___14. listened to my lungs in at least four places (mild bilateral expiratory wheezes audible).

___15. listened to my heart in at least three places (normal heart examination).

Communication Skills. The Examinee:

___16. explained asthma in words that a 17-year-old could understand.

___17. explained every step of the physical examination as it was being done.

___18. explained about the treatment needed (nebulizer, oxygen).

___19. began treating me for the breathing difficulty at the start of the test station.

___20. explained the purpose of the peak flowmeter.

___21. explained that I would stay in the office for a short time and then be able to go home.

___22. told me my mother has been called and is coming to the emergency room.

___23. explained that I would learn how to treat my asthma at home with medication pumps.

___24. relieved my anxiety about not being able to play sports or participate in gym class again.

___25. did not give me more information than I could handle.

___26. put me at ease.

If you performed 19 of these 26 tasks, you passed this test station.

You have 10 minutes to complete your patient note.

HISTORY—Include significant positives and negatives from the history of present illness, past medical history, review of systems, and social and family history.

_____
_____
_____
_____
_____
_____
_____
_____
_____
_____

PHYSICAL EXAMINATION—Indicate only the pertinent positive and negative findings related to the patient's chief complaint.

_____
_____
_____
_____
_____
_____
_____
_____
_____
_____

DIFFERENTIAL DIAGNOSIS—In order of likelihood, write no more than five differential diagnoses for this patient's current problems.

1. _____
2. _____
3. _____
4. _____
5. _____

DIAGNOSTIC WORKUP—Immediate plans for no more than five diagnostic studies.

1. _____
2. _____
3. _____
4. _____
5. _____

A SATISFACTORY PATIENT NOTE

HISTORY—Include significant positives and negatives from the history of present illness, past medical history, review of systems, and social and family history.

Ms. Jane Jett is a 17-year-old high school senior who was brought to the emergency room by the school nurse. The patient developed shortness of breath while running in gym class 2 hours ago. Ms. Jett states that similar episodes of shortness of breath have occurred while she was playing basketball and running to class, but the episodes resolved in an hour. The patient has some mild chest tightness but denies cough. She has not been ill recently with a URI and has no past medical history. She takes no medications and does not smoke cigarettes or use illicit drugs. She has no history of rashes or allergies. Asthma does not run in her family.

PHYSICAL EXAMINATION—Indicate only the pertinent positive and negative findings related to the patient's chief complaint.

The patient is a concerned and frightened teenager in mild respiratory distress.
T = 98.6°F. BP = 100/70 mmHg. RR = 28 breaths/min. HR = 100 beats/min. Oxygen saturation = 99% on room air. Able to speak in complete sentences.
HEENT: No use of accessory muscles. No nasal flaring.
Lungs: Positive for bilateral expiratory wheezes. Normal dullness and fremitus.
Heart: Normal S_1 and S_2.
Extremities: No edema or cyanosis.

DIFFERENTIAL DIAGNOSIS	DIAGNOSTIC WORKUP
In order of likelihood, write no more than five differential diagnoses for this patient's current problems.	Immediate plans for no more than five diagnostic studies.
1. asthma	1. peak flowmeter
2. pneumonia	2. CBC
3. cystic fibrosis	3. CXR
4. pulmonary embolus	4. pulmonary function tests
5. pneumothorax	5.

LEARNING OBJECTIVE FOR JANE JETT
EDUCATE A TEENAGER ABOUT HIS OR HER DISEASE

Jane Jett presents with an asthmatic episode. The breathing difficulty and chest tightness are frightening symptoms for this teenager. The physician taking care of Jane must be aware of her fear and quickly try to put her at ease. Good rapport between adolescent and physician is vital to obtaining an accurate history. Every step of the physical examination should be explained to the teenager to alleviate her fear and embarrassment. All equipment and monitoring devices, including the purpose of the peak flowmeter, should be explained in terms that are reassuring and understandable.

During the interview, Jane Jett recalls previous episodes of shortness of breath with exercise that, in retrospect, were her first exacerbations of asthma. The present episode occurred with exertion as well. Exercise is the most likely trigger for Jane Jett's asthmatic attacks (exercise-induced asthma).

The patient has no family history of asthma and takes no medications that may have caused asthma. She has no history of medical problems, i.e., cystic fibrosis. A history of allergies and rashes is denied by the patient, so an atopic condition is unlikely. She denies having a cough and is afebrile, so it is doubtful that respiratory infection is responsible for her symptoms.

On physical examination, the patient has bilateral scattered expiratory wheezes and is in mild respiratory distress. The heart examination is normal. There is no accessory muscle use and there is no nasal flaring. The patient is able to speak in full sentences without difficulty. She is experiencing a mild asthmatic episode. After a single inhalation of a β-adrenergic agonist, Ms. Jett becomes asymptomatic and her lungs on reexamination become clear to auscultation. While speaking to the patient and obtaining the history, the physician should have treated the acute exacerbation of asthma (all of the necessary items were in the examination room) to relieve the patient's symptoms and distress.

The patient will need instruction on using the medication pumps and the peak flowmeter at home. Teaching Jane Jett and her family about her disease and the triggers that may cause exacerbations requires continuous education and follow-up as an outpatient. The teenager should be told to breathe through her nose when exercising, which will humidify and filter the air. The young patient will be able to remain active using a cromolyn inhaler (70 percent of such patients will respond to this alone) as prophylaxis before gym class.

Patient Note Pearl: The **differential diagnosis** for shortness of breath includes asthma, pneumonia, upper airway obstruction, cystic fibrosis, congestive heart failure, bronchiolitis, pulmonary embolus, and pneumothorax. The **diagnostic workup** may include pulmonary function tests (FEV_1 will decline with exercise), and oxygen saturation. CBC, CXR, and an arterial blood gas (ABG) test should be ordered if infection or hypoxemia is suspected.

NOTES

Case 29

Jenny Jones is a 31-year-old schoolteacher who presents to the emergency room with an inability to "catch her breath."

Vital Signs:

Temperature	98.6°F orally
Blood pressure	120/90 mmHg
Respiratory rate	24 breaths per minute
Heart rate	100 beats per minute

On entering the examination room, you notice an anxious young woman who is able to speak only in short sentences. She has a tall, thin body habitus.

Examinee's Tasks

1. Obtain a focused and relevant history.
2. Perform a focused and relevant physical examination.
3. Discuss your initial diagnostic impressions with the patient.
4. Discuss follow-up tests with the patient.
5. After seeing the patient, complete paperwork relevant to the case.

MY CHECKLIST

History of Present Illness. The Examinee:

1. _____
2. _____
3. _____
4. _____
   _____
5. _____
6. _____
7. _____
8. _____
9. _____
   _____
10. _____
11. _____
12. _____
13. _____
14. _____
15. _____
16. _____
17. _____

Physical Examination. The Examinee:

18. _____
19. _____
20. _____
21. _____
22. _____

Communication Skills. The Examinee:

23. _____
24. _____
25. _____
    _____
26. _____

SP CHECKLIST FOR JENNY JONES

History of Present Illness. The Examinee:
___ 1. asked about the onset of the shortness of breath ("It started 12 hours ago.")
___ 2. asked what I was doing at the time the shortness of breath started ("Just watching television.")
___ 3. asked about problems with shortness of breath before ("Never.")
___ 4. asked about chest pain ("I do feel an achy kind of pain in my right chest; I thought I might have pulled a muscle.")
___ 5. asked about level of pain from 1 to 10 ("The pain is a 9. It's pretty intense.")
___ 6. asked about quality of pain (i.e., sharp or dull) ("The pain is very sharp.")
___ 7. asked whether the pain radiated ("Yes, it goes to my back.")
___ 8. asked whether pain was constant or intermittent ("The pain is constant.")
___ 9. asked whether the pain was worse with breathing ("Yes, the pain gets worse with deep breaths and even if I move a little.")
___10. asked about cough ("No.")
___11. asked about past medical history ("I've never been sick before.")
___12. asked about tobacco use ("Never.")
___13. asked about illicit drug use ("No.")
___14. asked about physical activity ("I run 2 miles every day.")
___15. asked about family history of lung problems ("No.")
___16. asked about recent trauma ("No.")
___17. asked about any leg pain ("No.")

Physical Examination. The Examinee:
___18. examined my trachea (trachea is midline)
___19. listened to my lungs in at least four places (diminished air entry over entire right side of chest).
___20. palpated my chest (no chest wall tenderness).
___21. listened to my heart in at least three places (normal heart examination).
___22. checked my calves for swelling and tenderness (none).

Communication Skills. The Examinee:
___23. explained every step of the physical examination as it was being done.
___24. explained the possible diagnoses (pneumothorax, pulmonary embolus, pneumonia).
___25. explained about the workup needed (chest radiograph, pulse oximetry or arterial blood gas, electrocardiogram).
___26. did not give me more information than I could handle.

If you performed 19 of these 26 tasks, you passed this test station.

You have 10 minutes to complete your patient note.

HISTORY—Include significant positives and negatives from the history of present illness, past medical history, review of systems, and social and family history.

_____

_____

_____

_____

_____

_____

_____

_____

_____

_____

PHYSICAL EXAMINATION—Indicate only the pertinent positive and negative findings related to the patient's chief complaint.

_____

_____

_____

_____

_____

_____

_____

_____

_____

_____

DIFFERENTIAL DIAGNOSIS—In order of likelihood, write no more than five differential diagnoses for this patient's current problems.

1. _____

2. _____

3. _____

4. _____

5. _____

DIAGNOSTIC WORKUP—Immediate plans for no more than five diagnostic studies.

1. _____

2. _____

3. _____

4. _____

5. _____

A SATISFACTORY PATIENT NOTE

HISTORY—Include significant positives and negatives from the history of present illness, past medical history, review of systems, and social and family history.

Ms. Jenny Jones is a 31-year-old schoolteacher who presents to the emergency room reporting an inability to catch her breath for the preceding 12 hours. The shortness of breath started at rest while she was sitting on the sofa watching television. She has an achy kind of right-sided chest pain that feels like a bad pulled muscle. On a scale of 1 to 10 the chest pain is a 9. The pain is sharp and radiates to her back. It is constant and gets worse with deep breathing or movement. She denies cough and previous illnesses. She considers herself to be a very healthy person and runs 2 miles every day. She does not smoke cigarettes or use illicit drugs. She has no family history of breathing or lung problems. She denies any recent trauma and has no leg pain.

PHYSICAL EXAMINATION—Indicate only the pertinent positive and negative findings related to the patient's chief complaint.

The patient is anxious and able to speak only in short sentences before having to catch her breath. She is holding the right side of her chest and appears to be in moderate respiratory distress. She has a tall and thin body habitus.
T = 98.6°F. BP = 120/90 mmHg. RR = 24 breaths/min.
HR = 100 beats/min.
HEENT: Trachea is midline.
Lungs: No chest wall tenderness. Diminished breath sounds over right posterior and anterior chest. No wheezes, rales, or rhonchi.
Heart: Normal S_1 and S_2. No rubs, murmurs, or gallops. No tachycardia.
Extremities: No cyanosis. No edema or calf tenderness. Negative Homans' sign.

DIFFERENTIAL DIAGNOSIS
In order of likelihood, write no more than five differential diagnoses for this patient's current problems.

1. pneumothorax
2. pulmonary embolus
3. pneumonia
4.
5.

DIAGNOSTIC WORKUP
Immediate plans for no more than five diagnostic studies.

1. CXR
2. pulse oximetry reading or ABG
3. electrocardiogram
4. bilateral lower extremity venous Dopplers
5. spiral CT scan or V/Q scan

LEARNING OBJECTIVE FOR JENNY JONES
RECOGNIZE A PATIENT PRESENTING WITH SPONTANEOUS PNEUMOTHORAX

Pain and dyspnea due to spontaneous pneumothorax often occur at rest; symptoms range from mild to severe and resolve within 24 hours even if the pneumothorax persists. Primary pneumothorax (no underlying lung disease or history of trauma) affects mainly tall, thin males between 10 and 30 years of age. Women, however, may still be affected. Family history and tobacco use are important contributing factors. Arterial blood gas or pulse oximetry reading may reveal hypoxemia and electrocardiogram may produce QRS axis and precordial T-wave changes. Chest radiograph reveals a pleural line but may be seen only on an expiratory film.

Physical Examination Pearl: Tension pneumothorax should be suspected in a patient who presents with marked tachycardia, hypotension, and mediastinal or tracheal deviation.

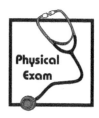

Patient Note Pearl: Occasionally a pneumothorax may mimic a myocardial infarction, pneumonia, or pulmonary embolus. The **workup** includes pulse oximetry or arterial blood gas, chest radiograph, and cardiothoracic or surgical consult. Patients who smoke should be advised to discontinue. Future exposure to high altitudes, scuba diving, and flying in unpressurized aircraft should be avoided.

Case 30

A mother has brought in her 4-month-old infant for a scheduled health maintenance visit.

Vital Signs:

Temperature	98.6°F
Blood pressure	105/60 mmHg
Respiratory rate	24 breaths per minute
Heart rate	100 beats per minute

Examinee's Tasks

1. Obtain a focused and relevant history.

2. Discuss your initial plan with the mother.

3. Provide education.

4. After seeing the patient, complete paperwork relevant to the case.

MY CHECKLIST

History of Present Illness. The Examinee:

1. _____
2. _____
   _____
3. _____
4. _____
   _____
5. _____
6. _____
7. _____
8. _____
9. _____
10. _____

Communication Skills. The Examinee:

11. _____
12. _____
13. _____
14. _____
15. _____
16. _____
17. _____
18. _____
19. _____

SP CHECKLIST FOR JOHNNY WILSON

History of Present Illness. The Examinee:

___ 1. started with an open-ended question, i.e., "How is everything going?" ("No problems, Doctor.")
___ 2. asked about the birth history of the baby, i.e., prenatal infections (none), method of delivery (NSVD), birth weight (7 pounds, 6 ounces), birth complications (none).
___ 3. asked about any recent illnesses ("None, thank goodness.")
___ 4. asked about the infant's eating habits ("Seems to be hungry all the time; I'm breast-feeding. I plan to breast-feed until he is 1 year old.")
___ 5. asked about the infant's sleeping habits ("Wakes up once a night to feed.")
___ 6. asked about the infant's hearing ("He seems to turn when he hears me speaking to him.")
___ 7. asked about the infant's vision ("He follows me around with his eyes.")
___ 8. checked on the infant's language development ("Infant coos and laughs.")
___ 9. asked about immunizations ("I took him for immunizations at 2 months.")
___10. asked if I was using the appropriate car seat ("Oh, most definitely.")

Communication Skills. The Examinee:

___11. stated that immunization would be needed for diphtheria, tetanus, and pertussis (DTP).
___12. stated that immunization would be needed for oral polio vaccine (OPV).
___13. stated that immunization would be needed for *Haemophilus influenzae* type b (Hib).
___14. discussed injury prevention with me, i.e., falls and choking.
___15. reinforced the positive things I was doing, i.e., "You really seem to be doing great."
___16. allowed me sufficient opportunity to ask questions.
___17. explained everything without using medical jargon.
___18. solicited my concerns.
___19. scheduled the 6-month visit.

If you performed 14 of these 19 tasks, you passed this test station.

You have 10 minutes to complete your patient note.

HISTORY—Include significant positives and negatives from the history of present illness, past medical history, review of systems, and social and family history.

_____
_____
_____
_____
_____
_____
_____
_____
_____
_____

PHYSICAL EXAMINATION—Indicate only the pertinent positive and negative findings related to the patient's chief complaint.

_____
_____
_____
_____
_____
_____
_____
_____
_____
_____

DIFFERENTIAL DIAGNOSIS—In order of likelihood, write no more than 5 differential diagnoses for this patient's current problems.

1. _____
2. _____
3. _____
4. _____
5. _____

DIAGNOSTIC WORKUP—Immediate plans for no more than five diagnostic studies.

1. _____
2. _____
3. _____
4. _____
5. _____

A SATISFACTORY PATIENT NOTE

HISTORY—Include significant positives and negatives from the history of present illness, past medical history, review of systems, and social and family history.

The mother of a 4-month-old is bringing in her infant for a scheduled health maintenance examination. The infant had no prenatal infections and his was an uncomplicated, normal, spontaneous vaginal delivery. His birth weight was 7 pounds, 6 ounces. Little Johnny Wilson has been healthy since birth. He is eating well and wakes once a night to feed. Other than the one feeding, he sleeps through the night. She plans to continue breast-feeding until he is 1 year old. The mother feels that the infant hears well, since he turns his head toward sounds and voices. He follows people with his eyes, so the mother feels he is able to see well. He coos and laughs and seems to be developing his language skills. The mother states that he last received immunizations at 2 months of age. He has not been ill. She always puts him in the appropriate child seat when in the car.

DIFFERENTIAL DIAGNOSIS
In order of likelihood, write no more than five differential diagnoses for this patient's current problems.

1. normal health maintenance visit
2. normal growth and development
3.
4.
5.

DIAGNOSTIC WORKUP
Immediate plans for no more than five diagnostic studies.

1. weight
2. height
3. head circumference
4. thorough physical examination
5.

LEARNING OBJECTIVE FOR JOHNNY WILSON
MONITOR GROWTH AND DEVELOPMENT IN A CHILD

Health maintenance visits for children are scheduled at regular intervals. In the first 2 years of life, the child should be seen by the pediatrician at 1, 2, 4, 6, 12, 15, 18, and 24 months of age. Laboratory testing and immunizations are performed at the appropriate intervals. Growth and development is followed at each visit by checking the child's weight, height, and head circumference. The physician should inquire about the child's pattern of sleep and diet (solid food may be started at 6 months of age). Monitoring the developmental progress of the child includes a careful assessment of the child's behavior, language, and motor skills.

The physical examination during health maintenance visits should be thorough and complete. Heart rate and blood pressure should be taken and the skin examined for lesions. Examination of the fontanelles should reveal closure by 18 months of age (the posterior fontanelle is usually closed by 8 weeks of age). The eyes should be examined for cataracts or infection. The ears should be investigated for otitis media. Anterior and posterior auscultation of the heart and lungs is necessary to elicit murmurs and assess for bilateral breath sounds. The abdomen should be palpated for masses and organomegaly. An examination of the extremities, with special attention to the hips, and a neurologic assessment—including the examination of cranial nerves, reflexes, and motor and sensory systems—are included in every health maintenance visit.

Health maintenance visits give the parents and the physician a chance to develop a relationship that will be helpful and educational to the parents (anticipatory guidance) and rewarding to the physician. The pediatrician should solicit questions and concerns from the parents and offer positive reinforcement, support, and reassurance when appropriate. A physician should assist parents to provide a safe and comfortable environment for children. Discussions about nutrition, exercise, dental care, and discipline should be part of the routine health maintenance visit.

History-Taking Pearl: Know the landmarks for normal development:

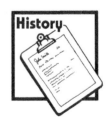

1 month: smiles, turns head, watches a person, holds chin up
2 months: recognizes parents, smiles on social contact, listens to voice, coos
3 months: laughs, listens to music, recognizes objects, reaches for objects and brings them to mouth
5 months: babbles, rolls over, prefers mother, lifts head
8 months: single words
10 months: sits up alone, plays peek-a-boo, waves bye-bye, grasps objects with thumb and forefinger, points to a desired object

12 months: two-word sentences, walks with one hand held, releases object to other person on request, plays simple ball game
17 months: conversational

Patient Note Pearl: Be able to discuss the immunization schedule with a new parent.

At birth: hepatitis B virus (HBV) [if mother's hepatitis B surface antigen (HBsAg) status is positive or unknown]
1 month: HBV
2 months: diphtheria, tetanus and pertussis vaccine (DTP), *H. influenzae* b conjugate vaccine (HbCV), and oral polio vaccine (OPV)
4 months: DTP, HbCV, and OPV
6 months: DTP, HBV, and HbCV
15 months: measles, mumps, rubella (MMR), HbCV, DTP, and OPV
4 years old: DTP, OPV, and MMR
11 years old: MMR
14 years old: tetanus, diphtheria toxoid vaccine (Td)

HBV schedule varies, depending on HBsAg status of mother; if mother's status is negative, then vaccination of HBV may be given: anytime from birth–3 months followed by second HBV 1 month after the first and a third HBV vaccine anytime between 6 and 18 months of age.

NOTES

Case 31

Nineteen-year-old Kenneth Smith presents complaining of a urethral discharge for 2 days, which has been dripping continuously and staining his underwear. On genital examination, discharge can be expressed from the penis. Penis, epididymis, and testes are normal. No inguinal lymphadenopathy. Rectal examination is normal.

Vital Signs:

Temperature	98.6°F
Blood pressure	120/80 mmHg
Heart rate	72 beats per minute
Respiratory rate	14 breaths per minute

Examinee's Tasks
(Do Not Repeat Genital or Rectal Examinations)

1. Obtain a focused and relevant history.
2. Perform a focused and relevant physical examination.
3. Discuss your initial diagnostic impressions with the patient.
4. Discuss follow-up tests with the patient.
5. After seeing the patient, complete paperwork relevant to the case.

MY CHECKLIST

History of Present Illness. The Examinee:

1. _____
2. _____
3. _____
   _____
4. _____
5. _____
6. _____
7. _____
8. _____
9. _____
10. _____
11. _____
12. _____
13. _____
14. _____
15. _____

Physical Examination. The Examinee:

16. _____
17. _____

Communication Skills. The Examinee:

18. _____
19. _____
   _____
20. _____
21. _____
22. _____
23. _____
24. _____
25. _____

SP CHECKLIST FOR KENNETH SMITH

History of Present Illness. The Examinee:

___ 1. asked about the color of the discharge ("Yellow-green.")

___ 2. asked about any blood in the discharge ("No.")

___ 3. asked about the quality of the burning on urination ("Yes, my urine does burn especially at the beginning of the flow.")

___ 4. asked about last sexual intercourse ("One week ago.")

___ 5. asked about any change in sexual function ("None.")

___ 6. asked about safe sexual practices ("I sometimes use a condom but I didn't a week ago.")

___ 7. asked about number of sexual partners over the last year ("Seven.")

___ 8. asked about any past medical history of sexually transmitted diseases ("None.")

___ 9. asked about sexual preferences ("I only have sex with women.")

___10. asked about any fevers or chills ("No.")

___11. asked about rashes ("None.")

___12. asked about any joint problems ("None.")

___13. asked about pain or swelling in the groin area ("No.")

___14. asked about any changes in his penis or testes ("No.")

___15. asked if I had any allergies to antibiotics, i.e., penicillin ("No.")

Physical Examination. The Examinee:

___16. listened to my abdomen in at least 4 places (normal examination).

___17. pressed on my abdomen (positive for mild suprapubic tenderness on palpation).

Communication Skills. The Examinee:

___18. washed hands before physical examination.

___19. discussed the differential diagnosis with me (gonorrhea, chlamydia, sexually transmitted disease, urinary tract infection).

___20. discussed plan with me (complete blood count, urethral culture, urinalysis).

___21. discussed treatment with me (antibiotics).

___22. informed me that my sexual partner would need to be examined and treated.

___23. was not judgmental.

___24. explained the importance of safe sexual practices.

___25. discussed the possibility of being tested for other sexually transmitted diseases (i.e., HIV, hepatitis, syphilis).

If you performed 18 of these 25 tasks, you passed this test station.

You have 10 minutes to complete your patient note.

HISTORY—Include significant positives and negatives from the history of present illness, past medical history, review of systems, and social and family history.

_____
_____
_____
_____
_____
_____
_____
_____
_____
_____
_____

PHYSICAL EXAMINATION—Indicate only the pertinent positive and negative findings related to the patient's chief complaint.

_____
_____
_____
_____
_____
_____
_____
_____
_____
_____
_____

DIFFERENTIAL DIAGNOSIS—In order of likelihood, write no more than five differential diagnoses for this patient's current problems.

1. _____
2. _____
3. _____
4. _____
5. _____

DIAGNOSTIC WORKUP—Immediate plans for no more than five diagnostic studies.

1. _____
2. _____
3. _____
4. _____
5. _____

A SATISFACTORY PATIENT NOTE

HISTORY—Include significant positives and negatives from the history of present illness, past medical history, review of systems, and social and family history.

Mr. Kevin Smith, 19 years old, has a 2-day history of urethral discharge that is dripping continuously staining his underwear. The discharge is yellowish green in color. There is no blood in the discharge. He has burning on urination, especially at the beginning of his stream. He denies fever, chills, rashes, and joint problems. He is a sexually active heterosexual who sometimes uses condoms. He has had seven sexual partners in the last year. His last sexual intercourse was with a new partner 1 week ago and he did not use a condom. His sexual function has been fine and he has not noticed any changes in his penis or testes. He has no history of sexually transmitted disease. He has no swelling in the groin area. He has no allergies to medications.

PHYSICAL EXAMINATION—Indicate only the pertinent positive and negative findings related to the patient's chief complaint.

Vital signs normal. Afebrile. He is a well-developed male in NAD but appears to be concerned and anxious.
Lungs: Clear to auscultation.
Heart: Normal S_1 and S_2.
Abdomen: Normal BS. Mild suprapubic tenderness. No rebound or CVA tenderness.
Genital Exam: Positive greenish brown nonbloody discharge. No lymphadenopathy. Normal penis, epididymis, and testes.
Rectal Exam: Normal examination.

DIFFERENTIAL DIAGNOSIS
In order of likelihood, write no more than five differential diagnoses for this patient's current problems.

1. urethritis from *Neisseria gonorrhoeae*
2. urethritis from *Chlamydia trachomatis*
3. urinary tract infection
4.
5.

DIAGNOSTIC WORKUP
Immediate plans for no more than five diagnostic studies.

1. CBC
2. urethral cultures
3. urinalysis
4. immunofluorescent slide test for *Chlamydia*
5. RPR or VDRL, HIV test

LEARNING OBJECTIVE FOR KENNETH SMITH
EVALUATE URETHRAL DISCHARGE IN A MALE

Urethral discharge is the most common symptom of sexually transmitted diseases. Possible organisms include *Neisseria gonorrhoeae, Chlamydia trachomatis, Gardnerella vaginalis, Trichomonas,* and *Candida.* Reiter's disease (urethritis, conjunctivitis, and arthritis) may mimic gonorrhea or coexist with it. The discharge of urethritis is thick and is usually yellow or brown in color. Dysuria and urethral itching may accompany the discharge. Systemic symptoms such as fever, chills, rash, and joint involvement may be seen when there is dissemination of the primary site of gonococci via the bloodstream. Bloody discharge suggests urethral carcinoma. Prevention is based on education and prophylaxis; condoms can reduce the risk of infection. Patients should be counseled in a nonjudgmental manner to practice safe sex in the future. Sexual partners must be examined and treated. Examinees should advise patients to be tested for other sexually transmitted diseases.

Patient Note Pearl: The differential diagnosis includes urethritis from *N. gonorrhoeae, C. trachomatis, G. vaginalis,* and *Trichomonas.* The plan should include a CBC, urinalysis, urethral cultures, immunofluorescent slide test for *Chlamydia,* and treatment of the sexual partner. Tests to evaluate for syphilis, HIV, and hepatitis may also be considered.

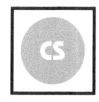

Case 32

Mr. Otto Lute is a 59-year-old man referred to the clinic from the emergency room, where he was seen the night before for shortness of breath. He was treated with diuretics and oxygen, improved, and was sent home.

Vital Signs:

Temperature	98.8°F
Blood pressure	150/90 mmHg
Heart rate	70 beats per minute
Respiratory rate	18 breaths per minute

Examinee's Tasks

1. Obtain a focused and relevant history.
2. Perform a focused and relevant physical examination.
3. Discuss your initial diagnostic impressions with the patient.
4. Discuss follow-up tests with the patient.
5. After seeing the patient, complete paperwork relevant to the case.

MY CHECKLIST

History of Present Illness. The Examinee:

1. _____
2. _____
   _____
3. _____
4. _____
5. _____
6. _____
   _____
7. _____
   _____
8. _____
9. _____
10. _____
11. _____
12. _____
13. _____
14. _____
15. _____
16. _____
17. _____

Physical Examination. The Examinee:

18. _____
19. _____
20. _____
21. _____
22. _____
23. _____
24. _____

Communication Skills. The Examinee:

25. _____
   _____
26. _____
27. _____
28. _____
29. _____

SP CHECKLIST FOR OTTO LUTE

History of Present Illness. The Examinee:

___ 1. asked about the onset of the breathing difficulty ("In all honesty, it started about 6 weeks ago.")
___ 2. asked about the progression of the shortness of breath ("Has progressively worsened over the 6 weeks; I couldn't take it anymore, so last night I went to the emergency room.")
___ 3. asked about aggravating factors("Gets worse with exertion and when I lie flat.")
___ 4. asked about any alleviating factors ("Gets better when I sit up and prop myself up.")
___ 5. asked about any cough ("Yes, especially at night; I sometimes can't sleep because of the annoying cough.")
___ 6. asked about any leg swelling ("Yes, my ankles are sometimes swollen; could that be from standing all day at my job as a security guard?")
___ 7. asked about having to sleep on more than one pillow ("Yes, I have been sleeping on three or four pillows recently; I can't seem to sleep lying flat like in the past.")
___ 8. asked about waking up in the middle of the night short of breath ("Yes; that was happening to me.")
___ 9. asked about any past medical history ("High blood pressure for 5 years.")
___10. asked about medications ("Yes, I am supposed to take diltiazam long-acting 120 mg once a day.")
___11. asked about compliance with medication ("Sometimes I forget to take the medication.")
___12. asked about diet ("I do eat a lot of salt, even though my old doctor told me to avoid salt.")
___13. asked about a history of chest pain ("None.")
___14. asked about a history of palpitations ("None.")
___15. asked about a history of dizziness ("No.")
___16. asked about tobacco use ("No.")
___17. asked about alcohol use ("None.")

Physical Examination. The Examinee:

___18. looked at my neck veins (no jugular venous distention noted).
___19. listened over my neck arteries (no carotid bruits).
___20. palpated the heart area for point of maximum pulsation.
___21. examined the heart in at least four places(no murmurs or gallops audible).
___22. listened to the lungs in at least four places (normal breath sounds).
___23. checked my liver size by tapping on it (liver size 12 cm in MCL).
___24. examined the legs for edema (no swelling).

Communication Skills. The Examinee:

___25. explained the initial diagnostic possibilities to me (i.e., congestive heart failure, hypertension-related heart disease).
___26. explained the next step in the plan (electrocardiogram and echocardiogram).
___27. explained that I must always take my medication for high blood pressure.
___28. explained that I must follow a low-salt diet.
___29. explained that an echocardiogram was a noninvasive test to look at the heart valves and the function of the heart.

If you performed 21 of these 29 tasks, you passed this test station.

You have 10 minutes to complete your patient note.

HISTORY—Include significant positives and negatives from the history of present illness, past medical history, review of systems, and social and family history.

_____

_____

_____

_____

_____

_____

_____

_____

_____

PHYSICAL EXAMINATION—Indicate only the pertinent positive and negative findings related to the patient's chief complaint.

_____

_____

_____

_____

_____

_____

_____

_____

_____

DIFFERENTIAL DIAGNOSIS—In order of likelihood, write no more than five differential diagnoses for this patient's current problems.

1. _____

2. _____

3. _____

4. _____

5. _____

DIAGNOSTIC WORKUP—Immediate plans for no more than five diagnostic studies.

1. _____

2. _____

3. _____

4. _____

5. _____

A SATISFACTORY PATIENT NOTE

HISTORY—Include significant positives and negatives from the history of present illness, past medical history, review of systems, and social and family history.

Mr. Otto Lute is a 59-year-old man referred to the clinic from the emergency room, where he was seen the night before for shortness of breath. He was treated with diuretics and oxygen, improved after several hours in the ER, and was sent home. Mr. Lute states that his difficulties with breathing started 6 weeks ago. It became so hard to breathe yesterday that he decided to go the emergency room. The shortness of breath was aggravated by exertion and lying down flat. He was awakening at night gasping for air and coughing. The breathing seemed to improve when he propped himself up on four pillows. His past medical history is significant for hypertension, but he had been noncompliant with his diltiazam. He uses a lot of salt on his food even though a former physician told him to avoid salt. He denies chest pain, palpitations, and dizziness. He does not smoke cigarettes or drink alcohol. He has had occasional leg swelling, which he attributes to standing all day at his job as a security guard.

PHYSICAL EXAMINATION—Indicate only the pertinent positive and negative findings related to the patient's chief complaint.

T = 98.8°F. BP = 150/90 mmHg. HR = 70 beats/min. RR = 18 breaths/min.
The patient appears older than his stated age. He is in mild respiratory distress.
HEENT: No JVD. Carotid pulse normal. No bruits.
Lungs: Normal breath sounds. No wheezes, rhonchi, or rales.
Heart: PMI 5th ICS MCL. Normal S_1 and S_2.
No murmurs, rubs, or gallops.
Abdomen: Liver size 12 cm in MCL. Nontender.
Extremities: No edema. Pulses 2+.

DIFFERENTIAL DIAGNOSIS
In order of likelihood, write no more than five differential diagnoses for this patient's current problems.

1. congestive heart failure
2. hypertension
3.
4.
5.

DIAGNOSTIC WORKUP
Immediate plans for no more than five diagnostic studies.

1. electrocardiogram
2. echocardiogram
3. BNP level
4. electrolytes
5. TSH level

LEARNING OBJECTIVE FOR OTTO LUTE

EVALUATE A PATIENT WITH NEW CONGESTIVE HEART FAILURE (CHF)

Patients with left ventricular failure present with fatigue, exertional dyspnea, cough, orthopnea, paroxysmal nocturnal dyspnea, rales, gallop rhythm, and pulmonary venous congestion. Patients with right ventricular failure present with elevated venous pressure, hepatomegaly, and peripheral edema. Mr. Lute presented to the emergency room with signs of left and right heart failure and responded to diuretics and oxygen. The heart failure is most likely due to uncontrolled hypertension—causing hypertensive heart disease—and lack of compliance with medication and diet. In several trials, antihypertensive therapy, especially when directed against systolic blood pressure, was effective in reducing the incidence of new-onset heart failure by 40 to 60 percent. Other possible causes of new heart failure include valvular heart disease, myocarditis, myocardial infarction, arrhythmias, and alcohol or drug abuse. The most useful test would be an echocardiogram. This will reveal the size and function of the ventricles and atria. It will detect pericardial effusions, valvular abnormalities, and wall motion abnormalities suggestive of previous myocardial infarction. Other tests to consider include a CBC (anemia may cause CHF), TSH (thyroid disease may cause CHF), serum potassium level (patient received diuretics) and the sensitive "B type" natriuretic peptide (BNP), which is expressed in the ventricles and is elevated when ventricular filling pressures are high.

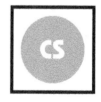

Patient Note Pearl: The **differential diagnosis** for this patient includes congestive heart failure, hypertensive heart disease, and, perhaps, myocardial infarction. The **diagnostic workup** may include a chest radiograph, electrocardiogram, cardiac isoenzymes, BNP level, and echocardiogram.

Case 33

Nineteen-month-old Baby Jane is brought to the emergency room by her nervous mother. The baby was in the playpen when she had a seizure that lasted approximately 5 minutes. The mother immediately rushed the child to the hospital. She is concerned that the baby may have meningitis.

Vital Signs:

Temperature	103.7°F rectally
Blood pressure	90/50 mmHg
Heart rate	146 beats per minute
Respiratory rate	26 breaths per minute

Examinee's Tasks

1. Obtain a focused and relevant history.

2. Discuss your initial diagnostic impressions with the mother.

3. Discuss follow-up tests with the mother.

4. After seeing the mother, complete paperwork relevant to the case.

MY CHECKLIST

History of Present Illness. The Examinee:

1. _____
2. _____
3. _____
   _____
4. _____
   _____
5. _____
6. _____
7. _____
8. _____
9. _____
10. _____
11. _____
12. _____
13. _____
14. _____
15. _____
16. _____

Communication Skills. The Examinee:

17. _____
    _____
18. _____
19. _____
20. _____
21. _____
22. _____
23. _____

SP CHECKLIST FOR BABY JANE

History of Present Illness. The Examinee:

___ 1. asked me to describe the seizure ("The entire body was shaking for 5 minutes.")

___ 2. asked about incontinence of the bladder or bowel ("Yes, she wet herself during the seizure.")

___ 3. asked what the baby was doing before the seizure, e.g., choking risks, such as eating, playing with a toy ("The baby was sleeping.")

___ 4. asked whether the baby was acting strangely after the seizure, i.e., postictally ("She seemed very different after the seizure; she seemed confused and agitated.")

___ 5. asked if the baby has a past medical history, e.g., retardation, neurologic problems, cerebral palsy ("No.")

___ 6. asked about any fever ("I didn't know she had a fever until now.")

___ 7. asked about any recent cough ("No.")

___ 8. asked about any gastrointestinal symptoms, i.e., vomiting or diarrhea ("No.")

___ 9. asked about any malodorous urine ("No.")

___10. asked about any recent rashes ("None.")

___11. asked if the baby had been irritable lately ("A little cranky for the last 2 days.")

___12. asked about the baby's appetite ("Not really eating very much lately.")

___13. asked about any recent immunization ("Immunizations are up to date; none recently.")

___14. asked about a family history of seizures ("No.")

___15. asked about ill contacts ("My other daughter had a cold recently, but she is better now.")

___16. asked about any recent history of trauma, falls, or ingestions ("No.")

Communication Skills. The Examinee:

___17. discussed the diagnosis (most likely a febrile seizure, which is common in childhood; meningitis, electrolyte imbalance less likely).

___18. explained that the seizure may recur.

___19. explained that this was not epilepsy.

___20. discussed the workup (blood work, urinalysis, observation).

___21. discussed the prognosis (very good).

___22. explained that the etiology is most likely viral or an early bacterial infection.

___23. addressed the mother's emotional concerns.

If you performed 17 of these 23 tasks, you passed this test station.

You have 10 minutes to complete your patient note.

HISTORY—Include significant positives and negatives from the history of present illness, past medical history, review of systems, and social and family history.

_____

_____

_____

_____

_____

_____

_____

_____

_____

_____

DIFFERENTIAL DIAGNOSIS—In order of likelihood, write no more than five differential diagnoses for this patient's current problems.

1. _____

2. _____

3. _____

4. _____

5. _____

DIAGNOSTIC WORKUP—Immediate plans for no more than five diagnostic studies.

1. _____

2. _____

3. _____

4. _____

5. _____

A SATISFACTORY PATIENT NOTE

HISTORY—Include significant positives and negatives from the history of present illness, past medical history, review of systems, and social and family history.

Baby Jane is a 19-month-old infant who, after having a 5-minute seizure, is brought to the emergency room by her mother. The infant was sleeping in her playpen when her entire body began to shake. Baby Jane wet herself during the seizure and was agitated afterwards. The baby has not been ill recently with fever, cough, diarrhea, or vomiting. She has had no malodorous urine or recent rashes. She has, however, been irritable for the last 2 days and seemed to have a poor appetite. Her immunizations are up to date and have not been recently given. There is no history of trauma, falls, or ingestions. The baby has no history of mental retardation, cerebral palsy, or neurologic disease. There is no family history of seizures. An older child has had a cold recently but is now asymptomatic.

DIFFERENTIAL DIAGNOSIS

In order of likelihood, write no more than five differential diagnoses for this patient's current problems.

1. febrile seizure
2. meningitis
3. electrolyte imbalance
4. accidental ingestion
5. hypoglycemia

DIAGNOSTIC WORKUP

Immediate plans for no more than five diagnostic studies.

1. CBC with differential
2. electrolytes
3. urinalysis
4. blood cultures
5. serum glucose level

LEARNING OBJECTIVE FOR BABY JANE
EVALUATE A CHILD WHO PRESENTS WITH A SEIZURE

Baby Jane presents to the emergency room after experiencing a single tonic-clonic seizure lasting 5 minutes while sleeping in her playpen. The mother's description of the episode (including the incontinence) and subsequent postictal period confirm the seizure diagnosis. Disorders that mimic seizures include breath-holding, narcolepsy, syncope, and shaking chills. Simple febrile seizures usually last less than 10 minutes and are followed by a postictal period. These seizures should be distinguished from complex febrile seizures, which recur over several hours or days and are focal and prolonged in duration. There is no previous history of seizure in this child, and the family history is unremarkable for seizures. The child has no existing predisposing condition for seizure, such as cerebral palsy, neurofibromatosis, or brain tumor. The incident was not preceded by cyanosis or choking. The mother denies trauma or accidental ingestion.

The temperature of 103.7°F rectally and the change in the child's personality (irritable, with loss of appetite) should concern the pediatrician. A source for the fever and possible bacteremia require a thorough interview and physical examination.

The mother denies any localizing symptoms to explain the fever, such as cough, vomiting, or diarrhea. There are no rashes or skin lesions consistent with a bacterial infection, viral exanthem, or other disease such as neurofibromatosis (café-au-lait spots). There have been no recent immunizations that could have caused the fever. A sibling recently recovered from a viral upper respiratory tract infection and should be considered an ill contact.

The child requires observation and antipyretics. A routine CT scan of the head is not indicated. Lumbar puncture is indicated in children with signs of meningitis or who present with complex febrile seizures, but a lumbar puncture has a low yield (<1 percent) in children with no signs of meningitis who present with simple febrile seizures.

The mother should be reassured by the physician that the fever causing the seizure is either viral in origin or an early sign of a bacterial infection, such as a pharyngitis or otitis media. The workup for this patient includes a leukocyte count and blood and urine cultures to search for occult bacteremia.

Inform the mother that febrile seizures are common in childhood and rarely lead to epilepsy (less than 1 percent lead to epilepsy, which is the same as the incidence in the general population). The mother should be aware that seizures may recur in up to one-third of children, usually within 2 years of the first episode. Anticonvulsants are not appropriate in uncomplicated febrile seizures.

Patient Note Pearl: The **differential diagnosis** for seizure in a child includes febrile seizure, infection (meningitis, encephalitis), electrolyte imbalance (hyponatremia), metabolic disorder (hypoglycemia), cyanosis from choking, heavy metal poisoning (lead), accidental ingestion of medication (theophylline, antihistamines, phenothiazines), other accidental ingestions, head trauma, and tumor. Seizure must be differentiated from shaking chills, breath-holding, syncope, and narcolepsy. The **diagnostic workup** may include CBC, electrolytes, serum glucose level, and, in selected patients, blood cultures, CT scan of the head, and lumbar puncture.

Case 34

Hillary Hanson is a 26-year-old graduate student, G0P0, menarche age 12, with normal menstrual periods, who has made an urgent appointment to see you because of severe lower abdominal pain.

Vital Signs:

Temperature	102.8°F rectally
Blood pressure	110/67 mmHg
Heart rate	96 beats per minute
Respiratory rate	16 breaths per minute

The nurse practitioner informs you that Ms. Hanson's pelvic examination was positive for right adnexal tenderness and a malodorous discharge.

Examinee's Tasks
(Do not repeat the gynecologic examination)

1. Obtain a focused and relevant history.
2. Perform a focused and relevant physical examination.
3. Discuss your initial diagnostic impressions with the patient.
4. Discuss follow-up tests with the patient.
5. After seeing the patient, complete paperwork relevant to the case.

MY CHECKLIST

History of Present Illness. The Examinee:

1. _____
2. _____
   _____
3. _____
4. _____
5. _____
6. _____
7. _____
8. _____
9. _____
10. _____
11. _____
12. _____
13. _____
14. _____
15. _____
16. _____

Physical Examination. The Examinee:

17. _____
18. _____
    _____
19. _____
20. _____
21. _____

Communication Skills. The Examinee:

22. _____
23. _____
24. _____
25. _____
    _____
26. _____
27. _____
28. _____

SP CHECKLIST FOR MS. HANSON

History of Present Illness. The Examinee:

___ 1. asked about the location of the pain ("Lower part of my abdomen.")
___ 2. asked about the onset of the pain ("It started 3 days ago after my menstrual period; it's not like my PMS though.")
___ 3. asked about the quality of the pain ("It is dull and constant.")
___ 4. asked about the intensity of the pain ("On a scale of 1 to 10, where 10 is the worst, this is an 8.")
___ 5. asked about any alleviating factors ("None. I tried ibuprofen and it didn't work.")
___ 6. asked about any aggravating factors ("Walking and moving make it worse.")
___ 7. asked about any association with nausea or vomiting ("No.")
___ 8. asked about a change in bowel movements, i.e., diarrhea or constipation ("No.")
___ 9. asked about any urinary complaints, i.e., hematuria, frequency, dysuria and nocturia ("No.")
___10. asked about fever ("I felt feverish but didn't take my temperature.")
___11. asked about vaginal discharge ("Yes; but it is probably the end of my menstrual period.")
___12. asked about sexual history ("I have had only one partner for the last 3 years and he is feeling fine.")
___13. asked about any sexually transmitted diseases ("None.")
___14. asked about history of pregnancy ("No; I have always used birth control pills.")
___15. asked about use of condoms ("No.")
___16. asked about last Pap smear ("Last year, and it was normal.")

Physical Examination. The Examinee:

___17. listened to my abdomen with a stethoscope (normal bowel sounds).
___18. asked about the appendectomy scar clearly visible with inspection of my abdomen ("I forgot to tell you I had an appendectomy.").
___19. palpated my abdomen (SP will complain of severe pain on right lower side).
___20. attempted to elicit rebound tenderness (positive rebound tenderness elicited on right lower side).
___21. tried to elicit costovertebral angle tenderness (none).

Communication Skills. The Examinee:

___22. discussed the initial impression with me [probable pelvic inflammatory disease (PID) or tubo-ovarian abscess].
___23. discussed the workup for this problem (blood work, antibiotics, pelvic examination, pelvic ultrasonography).
___24. explained that this could lead to infertility if not treated.
___25. explained that this was a sexually transmitted disease and her partner must use condoms in the future ("But my boyfriend is faithful to me; are you saying he's been with someone else?")
___26. explained that the sexual partner should be examined and treated.
___27. was empathetic.
___28. did not ignore or avoid my questions regarding my boyfriend's infidelity.

If you performed 20 of these 28 tasks, you passed this test station.

You have 10 minutes to complete your patient note.

HISTORY—Include significant positives and negatives from the history of present illness, past medical history, review of systems, and social and family history.

_____
_____
_____
_____
_____
_____
_____
_____
_____
_____

PHYSICAL EXAMINATION—Indicate only the pertinent positive and negative findings related to the patient's chief complaint.

_____
_____
_____
_____
_____
_____
_____
_____
_____
_____

DIFFERENTIAL DIAGNOSIS—In order of likelihood, write no more than five differential diagnoses for this patient's current problems.

1. _____
2. _____
3. _____
4. _____
5. _____

DIAGNOSTIC WORKUP—Immediate plans for no more than five diagnostic studies.

1. _____
2. _____
3. _____
4. _____
5. _____

A SATISFACTORY PATIENT NOTE

HISTORY—Include significant positives and negatives from the history of present illness, past medical history, review of systems, and social and family history.

Ms. Hillary Hanson is a 26-year-old graduate student, G0P0, who complains of a 3-day history of severe right-lower-quadrant abdominal pain. The pain started on day 3 of her menstrual period but it differs from her menstrual pain. It is dull and constant. On a scale of 1 to 10, the pain is an 8. Nothing seems to alleviate it (she tried ibuprofen) and it is made worse by walking or moving. She denies nausea, vomiting, constipation, and diarrhea. She has no frequency, dysuria, nocturia, or hematuria. She did not take her temperature but felt feverish the last several days. She has a malodorous vaginal discharge but thinks it is associated with her menses. She is monogamous and has been sexually active with one partner for 3 years. She has no history of sexually transmitted disease. Her partner does not use condoms. Her partner is asymptomatic. She uses oral contraceptives. Her last pap smear was 1 year ago and was normal.

PHYSICAL EXAMINATION—Indicate only the pertinent positive and negative findings related to the patient's chief complaint.

T = 102.8°F. BP = 110/67 mmHg. HR = 96 beats/min.
The patient is lying still on the stretcher. She is grimacing in pain and uncomfortable. She moves slowly. She is shy about answering sexual history questions but does so when asked directly.
Skin: Appendectomy scar present.
Lungs: Clear to auscultation.
Heart: Normal S_1 and S_2.
Abdomen: Normal BS. +RLQ tenderness. +RLQ rebound tenderness. No CVA tenderness.
Genital Examination: Cervical motion and right adnexal tenderness. Positive for a malodorous discharge.

DIFFERENTIAL DIAGNOSIS
In order of likelihood, write no more than five differential diagnoses for this patient's current problems.

1. pelvic inflammatory disease
2. tuboovarian abscess
3. ovarian cyst
4. ectopic pregnancy
5.

DIAGNOSTIC WORKUP
Immediate plans for no more than five diagnostic studies.

1. CBC with differential
2. pelvic sonogram
3. pregnancy test
4. vaginal culture
5. treat partner

LEARNING OBJECTIVE FOR MS. HANSON
APPROACH TO THE SEXUALLY ACTIVE WOMAN
WITH LOWER ABDOMINAL PAIN AND FEVER

Ms. Hanson presents with a 3-day history of severe right-lower-quadrant pain, which is dull and constant. She is febrile, with a temperature of 102.8°F. She uses birth control pills and would be at low risk for an ectopic pregnancy. Pyelonephritis is doubtful without urinary complaints and no costovertebral angle tenderness. Gastroenteritis is a consideration, but the patient denies having nausea, vomiting, and diarrhea. As the interview progresses, Ms. Hanson admits that she does not require the use of condoms because she has had a faithful sexual partner for 3 years.

On abdominal examination, Ms. Hanson is found to have a tender right-lower-quadrant and rebound tenderness. She has an appendectomy scar (even if the SP had been asked about previous surgery, she would have forgotten about the appendectomy until the scar was mentioned by the examinee during the physical examination). Pelvic examination was positive for a malodorous discharge and right adnexal tenderness. PID usually occurs after a menstrual period. Risk factors for the disease include multiple sexual partners and the use of an intrauterine contraceptive device. Hospitalization is required if the patient has a high temperature or if there is a possibility of a tuboovarian abscess. If untreated, PID may lead to infertility.

Ms. Hanson will ask her sexual partner to be examined and treated for sexually transmitted diseases. She will be educated and counseled regarding safe sexual practice including the boyfriend's use of condoms. Since the patient is very upset about her boyfriend's infidelity, the physician must be supportive and understanding.

Patient Note Pearl: The **differential diagnosis** for this patient includes PID, tuboovarian abscess, ectopic pregnancy, complicated ovarian cyst, and endometriosis. Appendicitis would have been included in the differential diagnosis, but the patient had had an appendectomy. The **diagnostic workup** includes CBC, a pregnancy test, pelvic sonography, and treatment of partner.

Case 35

You have provided gynecologic care for 50-year-old Holly Faithful for over 10 years. She is a healthy patient who has had normal Pap smears and mammograms in the past. Her last checkup with you was 11 months ago. She is complaining of episodes of diaphoresis, which she feels may be the "hot flashes" of menopause. You know her to have no past medical history and she takes no medications. She does not smoke, drink, or use drugs. Her sister, who was also your patient, died of breast cancer 2 years ago. Her vital signs are normal.

Examinee's Tasks

1. Obtain a focused and relevant history.
2. Discuss your initial diagnostic impressions with the patient.
3. Discuss follow-up tests with the patient.
4. Provide patient education.
5. After seeing the patient, complete paperwork relevant to the case.

MY CHECKLIST

History of Present Illness. The Examinee:

1. _____
2. _____
3. _____
4. _____
5. _____
   _____
6. _____
7. _____
8. _____
9. _____
   _____
10. _____
    _____

Communication Skills. The Examinee:

11. _____
12. _____
13. _____
14. _____
15. _____
16. _____
    _____
17. _____
18. _____

SP CHECKLIST FOR MRS. FAITHFUL

History of Present Illness. The Examinee:

___ 1.   asked about the onset of the hot flashes ("They started about 6 months ago.")

___ 2.   asked about the duration of the hot flashes ("They last about 5 minutes.")

___ 3.   asked about the frequency of the hot flashes ("They happen maybe 10 times a day.")

___ 4.   asked what alleviates the hot flashes ("It helps if I open a window or turn the air conditioner on.")

___ 5.   asked what aggravates the hot flashes ("Stress and the hot weather. They happen at night and wake me up from sleep.")

___ 6.   asked about my last menstrual period ("No menstrual period for 12 months.")

___ 7.   asked about any urinary problems, i.e., incontinence, frequency, dysuria ("No.")

___ 8.   asked about any vaginal dryness or itchiness ("Yes.")

___ 9.   asked about any dyspareunia ("Yes. My husband has been afraid to initiate intercourse with me because I complain of pain.")

___10.   asked about any feelings of anxiety or depression ("I am very anxious and on edge; I'm driving my husband crazy.")

Communication Skills. The Examinee:

___11.   explained that it was menopause (plausible diagnosis).

___12.   offered to help explain the situation to the husband.

___13.   discussed the use of a topical estrogen for vaginal dryness.

___14.   discussed the importance of calcium and vitamin D in the diet to prevent bone loss.

___15.   discussed the importance of exercise to prevent heart disease and osteoporosis.

___16.   discussed a special study to diagnose osteoporosis [bone densitometry or a dual energy x-ray absorptiometry scan (DEXA)].

___17.   discussed estrogen use with the strong family history of breast cancer.

___18.   suggested a support group in the community for additional discussion.

If you performed 13 of these 18 tasks, you passed this test.

You have 10 minutes to complete your patient note.

HISTORY—Include significant positives and negatives from the history of present illness, past medical history, review of systems, and social and family history.

_____
_____
_____
_____
_____
_____
_____
_____
_____
_____

DIFFERENTIAL DIAGNOSIS—In order of likelihood, write no more than five differential diagnoses for this patient's current problems.

1. _____
2. _____
3. _____
4. _____
5. _____

DIAGNOSTIC WORKUP—Immediate plans for no more than five diagnostic studies.

1. _____
2. _____
3. _____
4. _____
5. _____

A SATISFACTORY PATIENT NOTE

HISTORY—Include significant positives and negatives from the history of present illness, past medical history, review of systems, and social and family history.

Mrs. Holly Faithful is a 50-year-old woman with a 6-month history of hot flashes. She is having approximately 10 episodes a day. Each hot flash is 5 minutes in duration. She has noticed that the hot flashes tend to occur at night, waking her from sleep, and that stress and hot weather aggravate the episodes. The flashes are sometimes so intense that she must open a window or turn the air conditioner on to obtain relief. She denies incontinence, frequency, and dysuria. She admits to vaginal dryness and itchiness. She has dyspareunia; her husband is afraid to have sexual intercourse with her because of her pain. Mrs. Faithful feels anxious at times and is on edge. She is concerned that she might be "driving her husband crazy" and they are both wondering if she could be going through menopause. Her last menstrual period was 12 months ago. Mrs. Faithful has no past medical history and takes no medications. She does not smoke cigarettes, drink alcohol, or take illicit drugs. Family history is significant for a sister who died of breast cancer. Mrs. Faithful has had normal pap smears and mammograms. Her last mammogram was 11 months ago.

DIFFERENTIAL DIAGNOSIS

In order of likelihood, write no more than five differential diagnoses for this patient's current problems.

1. menopause (secondary amenorrhea)
2. vaginal dryness
3. dyspareunia
4.
5.

DIAGNOSTIC WORKUP

Immediate plans for no more than five diagnostic studies.

1. DEXA scan
2. yearly mammogram
3.
4.
5.

LEARNING OBJECTIVE FOR MRS. FAITHFUL

RECOGNIZE AND COUNSEL A PATIENT EXPERIENCING MENOPAUSE

Mrs. Faithful has been a healthy patient in your practice. At the age of 50, she is presenting with hot flashes and a 12-month history of secondary amenorrhea. Her husband is having difficulty coping with her mood swings and irritability. She is experiencing dyspareunia, which is making her husband aloof and distant. Her presentation is consistent with menopause.

Mrs. Faithful is experiencing a normal event in life and needs support and reassurance from her physician. She should be made aware of other symptoms of menopause, such as urinary frequency, dysuria, and incontinence. Patients may become depressed or anxious during this time, but there is no evidence that personality or mood changes are due to menopause.

A discussion about proper exercise and diet in the middle years will help prevent bone mineral loss and heart disease in such patients. The diet should be supplemented with 1000 mg of calcium and 200 to 400 units of vitamin D per day. Over-the-counter vaginal lubricants may help relieve vaginal dryness and dyspareunia. The gynecologist should offer to meet the husband to address his concerns about intimacy.

Hormone replacement therapy (HRT) requires careful discussion and consideration in a patient with a family history of breast cancer. Mrs. Faithful should be involved in every aspect of her care and in the estrogen replacement decision-making process. Other medications may be used for the hot flashes, such as α-adrenergic agonists (e.g., clonidine). Women with early menopause or those at high risk for osteoporosis can have bone mass quantitated by a DEXA scan. Patients with poor bone density may be managed with biphosphonates.

A support group may serve as an additional resource for Mrs. Faithful. She could enhance her knowledge of menopause and exchange experiences with similar women in her community.

Case 36

Mrs. Peggy Perky, 22 years old (G0P0), complains of the sudden onset of abdominal pain. The gynecologic examination is positive for some old blood in the vault and left adnexal tenderness; the uterus is slightly enlarged, mobile, and tender. No masses were palpated.

Vital Signs:

Temperature	98.6°F
Blood pressure	115/80 mmHg
Heart rate	110 beats per minute
Respiratory rate	12 breaths per minute

Examinee's Tasks
(Do not repeat the gynecologic examination)

1. Obtain a focused and relevant history.

2. Perform a focused and relevant physical examination.

3. Discuss your initial diagnostic impressions with the patient.

4. Discuss follow-up tests with the patient.

5. After seeing the patient, complete paperwork relevant to the case.

MY CHECKLIST

History of Present Illness. The Examinee:

1. _____
2. _____
3. _____
4. _____
5. _____
6. _____
7. _____
8. _____
9. _____
10. _____
11. _____
12. _____
13. _____
14. _____
15. _____
16. _____

Physical Examination. The Examinee:

17. _____
18. _____
19. _____
20. _____
21. _____

Communication Skills. The Examinee:

22. _____
    _____
23. _____
    _____
24. _____
25. _____

SP CHECKLIST FOR MRS. PERKY

History of Present Illness. The Examinee:

___ 1. asked about the location of the pain ("It's in the left lower part of my abdomen.")

___ 2. asked about the onset of the pain ("It started about 1 hour ago.")

___ 3. asked about the quality of the pain ("Stabbing and tearing.")

___ 4. asked about the intensity of the pain ("On a scale of 1 to 10, this is a 9.")

___ 5. asked about the progression of the pain ("It is getting worse as we speak.")

___ 6. asked about any aggravating factors ("Moving around.")

___ 7. asked about any alleviating factors ("Nothing really helps.")

___ 8. asked about any radiation of the pain ("It goes to my left shoulder and my neck.")

___ 9. asked about any urinary complaints ("No.")

___10. asked about my last menstrual period ("It was 7 weeks ago.")

___11. asked if I had had a pregnancy test ("No.")

___12. asked about any vaginal bleeding ("A small amount of bleeding after the pain started.")

___13. asked about any gastrointestinal complaints, i.e., vomiting or change in bowel movements ("No.")

___14. asked about my sexual history ("My husband has been my only sexual partner for 4 years; he is faithful.")

___15. asked about contraception ("No method of contraception used.")

___16. asked about my gynecologic history ("History of pelvic inflammatory disease 5 years ago.")

Physical Examination. The Examinee:

___17. checked my blood pressure lying down and sitting up or standing (positive orthostatic changes).

___18. listened to my abdomen with a stethoscope (positive bowel sounds).

___19. palpated gently on my abdomen (SP will complain of left-lower-quadrant pain).

___20. palpated my abdomen deeply (SP will complain of severe left-lower-quadrant pain).

___21. tried to elicit rebound tenderness (positive rebound tenderness).

Communication Skills. The Examinee:

___22. discussed the diagnostic possibilities with me (i.e., ectopic pregnancy, PID, tuboovarian abscess, ruptured luteal cyst).

___23. discussed the next step in management (blood work, pregnancy test, pelvic examination, intravenous fluids, sonogram).

___24. offered to speak to my husband and explain the situation.

___25. was aware of my discomfort during the physical examination.

If you performed 18 of these 25 tasks, you passed this test station.

You have 10 minutes to complete your patient note.

HISTORY—Include significant positives and negatives from the history of present illness, past medical history, review of systems, and social and family history.

_____
_____
_____
_____
_____
_____
_____
_____
_____
_____

PHYSICAL EXAMINATION—Indicate only the pertinent positive and negative findings related to the patient's chief complaint.

_____
_____
_____
_____
_____
_____
_____
_____
_____
_____

DIFFERENTIAL DIAGNOSIS—In order of likelihood, write no more than five differential diagnoses for this patient's current problems.

1. _____
2. _____
3. _____
4. _____
5. _____

DIAGNOSTIC WORKUP—Immediate plans for no more than five diagnostic studies.

1. _____
2. _____
3. _____
4. _____
5. _____

A SATISFACTORY PATIENT NOTE

HISTORY—Include significant positives and negatives from the history of present illness, past medical history, review of systems, and social and family history.

Mrs. Peggy Perky is a 22-year-old woman with the chief complaint of abdominal pain, which has lasted for 1 hour. She describes the pain as a 9 on a scale on 1 to 10. The abdominal pain is stabbing and tearing in nature and is located in the left lower quadrant. It has been progressively worsening and is now radiating to her left shoulder and neck. There are no alleviating factors and movement of any kind makes the pain worse. She denies dysuria, nausea, vomiting, or change in bowel movement. Her last period was 7 weeks ago but she noticed some small amount of vaginal bleeding after the abdominal pain started. She has not had a pregnancy test. She is monogamous with her husband of 4 years and does not use contraception. Past gynecologic history is significant for pelvic inflammatory disease 5 years ago.

PHYSICAL EXAMINATION—Indicate only the pertinent positive and negative findings related to the patient's chief complaint.

T = 98.6°F. RR = 12 breaths/min.
BP = 115/80 mmHg. HR = 110 beats/min lying down.
BP = 90/60 mmHg. HR = 120 beats/min with legs dangling.
The patient is a pale, anxious woman in distress due to abdominal pain.
Lungs: Clear to auscultation.
Heart: Normal S_1 and S_2.
Abdomen: +BS. Severe LLQ pain with palpation. +Rebound tenderness.
Gynecologic: Old blood in the vault. Closed os. Left adnexal tenderness. Uterus is slightly enlarged, mobile and tender. No masses palpable.

DIFFERENTIAL DIAGNOSIS

In order of likelihood, write no more than five differential diagnoses for this patient's current problems.

1. ectopic pregnancy
2. orthostasis
3. pelvic inflammatory disease
4. tuboovarian abscess
5. ruptured corpus luteum cyst

DIAGNOSTIC WORKUP

Immediate plans for no more than five diagnostic studies.

1. pregnancy test
2. CBC
3. pelvic sonogram
4. electrolytes
5. BUN and creatinine

LEARNING OBJECTIVE FOR MRS. PERKY
APPROACH TO THE SEXUALLY ACTIVE WOMAN
WITH LOWER ABDOMINAL PAIN AND SIGNS OF EARLY SHOCK

The patient presents with sudden onset of severe left-lower-quadrant pain that radiates to the shoulder not associated with gastrointestinal or urinary symptoms. She has some minimal vaginal bleeding that developed after the pain. She is afebrile but is hypotensive and tachycardic. Gynecologic examination is positive for blood, adnexal tenderness, and a slightly enlarged but mobile uterus. The most likely diagnosis is ectopic pregnancy. The pain and bleeding along with the history of amenorrhea, with no use of contraception, is consistent with this diagnosis. The past history of PID is a risk factor for ectopic pregnancy. Other risk factors for ectopic pregnancy include the use of an intrauterine device and a previous history of an ectopic pregnancy.

Tuboovarian abscess and PID must be included in the differential diagnosis (even if promiscuity is denied); but, in these cases, the patient would most likely be febrile and have no history of amenorrhea. A ruptured luteal cyst, like an ectopic pregnancy, may be present, but sonography (demonstrating the intrauterine pregnancy) will distinguish between these two problems.

The radiation of the pain to the shoulder is due to diaphragmatic irritation from hemoperitoneum. Examination of the abdomen reveals rebound tenderness. The "stat" pregnancy test will be positive in this patient.

Mrs. Perky will need pelvic ultrasonography to confirm the adnexal mass and the absence of an intrauterine pregnancy. Intravenous hydration and often blood transfusions are needed to correct hypotension and tachycardia. Surgery for the ruptured ectopic pregnancy is performed after the patient is stabilized.

Patient Note Pearl: The **differential diagnosis** for this patient includes ectopic pregnancy, tuboovarian abscess, PID, ruptured corpus luteal cyst, appendicitis, endometriosis, and kidney stone. The **diagnostic workup** includes pregnancy test (the urine pregnancy test may be negative but the serum β-human chorionic gonadotropin test will almost always be positive), CBC, and pelvic sonogram.

Case 37

You are asked to see Mrs. Stacy Stevens (G1P0). She is 24 years old and is 9 weeks pregnant. Her obstetrician, your partner, is attending a conference. The patient complains of vaginal bleeding and feels she may be having a miscarriage. The nurse practitioner has performed the gynecologic examination and tells you that the cervical os is closed and there is no effacement; uterus is 10 weeks in size; there is no blood, tissue, or discharge.

Vital Signs:

Temperature	98.6°F
Blood pressure	105/70 mmHg
Heart rate	80 beats per minute
Respiratory rate	12 breaths per minute

Examinee's Tasks
(Do not repeat the gynecologic examination)

1. Obtain a focused and relevant history.
2. Perform a focused and relevant physical examination.
3. Discuss your initial diagnostic impressions with the patient.
4. Discuss follow-up tests with the patient.
5. After seeing the patient, complete paperwork relevant to the case.

MY CHECKLIST

History of Present Illness. The Examinee:

1. _____
2. _____
   _____
3. _____
4. _____
5. _____
   _____
6. _____
7. _____
8. _____
9. _____
10. _____
11. _____

Physical Examination. The Examinee:

12. _____
13. _____

Communication Skills. The Examinee:

14. _____
    _____
15. _____
16. _____
17. _____
18. _____
19. _____
20. _____
21. _____
22. _____
23. _____

SP CHECKLIST FOR MRS. STEVENS

History of Present Illness. The Examinee:

___ 1. asked about the onset of the vaginal bleeding ("It started about 5 hours ago.")

___ 2. asked about the quantity of the vaginal bleeding, i.e., how many pads were soaked; is bleeding more or less than menstrual period? ("Just one pad, like the first day of my period, but I'm afraid.")

___ 3. asked about the progression of the bleeding ("I think it is slowing down; not getting any worse.")

___ 4. verified gestational age by asking the date of my last menstrual period ("Nine weeks ago.")

___ 5. asked if I had a sonogram ("Yes. The sonogram revealed a baby was in the uterus. I keep my prenatal appointments.")

___ 6. asked about any abdominal pain or cramps ("Some cramps, like my period.")

___ 7. asked what I was doing at the time the vaginal bleeding started ("Just watching television.")

___ 8. asked about sexual intercourse in the last 24 hours, i.e., could this be postcoital bleeding? ("No.")

___ 9. asked about any recent stress ("None. Everything has been great; my husband and I are so happy.")

___10. asked about any tobacco use ("No.")

___11. asked about any illicit drug use ("No.")

Physical Examination. The Examinee:

___12. listened to my abdomen with a stethoscope (normal bowel sounds auscultated).

___13. palpated gently on my abdomen (no tenderness elicited).

Communication Skills. The Examinee:

___14. explained the initial diagnostic possibilities to me (i.e., threatened abortion, incomplete abortion, postcoital bleeding).

___15. explained that this was a common problem early in pregnancy.

___16. explained the workup (pelvic examination and ultrasonography).

___17. explained that many women who experience first-trimester bleeding carry their pregnancy to term.

___18. advised bed rest for the next 48 hours.

___19. advised me to abstain from sexual intercourse for 1 week.

___20. told me to call immediately if further bleeding or cramps occurred.

___21. arranged for a follow-up appointment with me.

___22. offered to help discuss the problem with my husband.

___23. showed concern for me.

If you performed 17 of these 23 tasks, you passed this test station.

You have 10 minutes to complete your patient note.

HISTORY—Include significant positives and negatives from the history of present illness, past medical history, review of systems, and social and family history.

_____
_____
_____
_____
_____
_____
_____
_____
_____
_____
_____

PHYSICAL EXAMINATION—Indicate only the pertinent positive and negative findings related to the patient's chief complaint.

_____
_____
_____
_____
_____
_____
_____
_____
_____
_____

DIFFERENTIAL DIAGNOSIS—In order of likelihood, write no more than five differential diagnoses for this patient's current problems.

1. _____
2. _____
3. _____
4. _____
5. _____

DIAGNOSTIC WORKUP—Immediate plans for no more than five diagnostic studies.

1. _____
2. _____
3. _____
4. _____
5. _____

A SATISFACTORY PATIENT NOTE

HISTORY—Include significant positives and negatives from the history of present illness, past medical history, review of systems, and social and family history.

Mrs. Stacy Stevens (G1P0) is a 24-year-old woman who is in her ninth week of pregnancy. She is compliant with her prenatal care visits and her sonogram revealed a uterine pregnancy. She has come to the office because, for the last 5 hours, she has had vaginal bleeding. The bleeding started while she was watching television. The amount of bleeding is similar to the first day of menstrual flow (one pad). She states that the bleeding is accompanied by crampy abdominal pain similar to the pain of her periods. She denies sexual intercourse in the last 24 hours and is not under any stress. She does not smoke cigarettes or use illicit drugs. She thinks that the bleeding is not worsening and is slowing down.

PHYSICAL EXAMINATION—Indicate only the pertinent positive and negative findings related to the patient's chief complaint.

BP = 105/70 mmHg. HR = 80 beats/min. RR = 12. Afebrile.
Frightened and tearful young woman who is pleasant and cooperative.
Heart: Normal S_1 and S_2.
Lungs: Clear to auscultation.
Abdomen: Normal BS. Nontender. No rebound.
Gynecologic Exam: Cervical os closed. No effacement. Uterus 10 weeks in size. No blood, tissue, or discharge present.

DIFFERENTIAL DIAGNOSIS	DIAGNOSTIC WORKUP
In order of likelihood, write no more than five differential diagnoses for this patient's current problems.	Immediate plans for no more than five diagnostic studies.
1. threatened abortion	1. CBC
2. incomplete abortion	2. pelvic sonogram
3. complete abortion	3. pregnancy test
4. postcoital bleeding	4.
5. trophoblastic disease	5.

LEARNING OBJECTIVE FOR MRS. STEVENS
COUNSEL A PATIENT REGARDING FIRST-TRIMESTER VAGINAL BLEEDING

Mrs. Stevens has a minimal amount of vaginal bleeding during the first trimester of pregnancy. She is frightened that this is a sign of a miscarriage. She is not under any emotional stress and was not engaging in overactivity when the bleeding began. The bleeding is not due to other causes such as recent sexual intercourse (postcoital bleeding). The differential diagnosis for first-trimester bleeding includes threatened, incomplete, and complete abortion. Approximately 25 percent of women will have some bleeding early in pregnancy, which makes this problem a common complaint. The physician should verify the gestational age and inquire about a sonogram. Risk factors for miscarriage include tobacco and drug use.

First-trimester bleeding is often associated with crampy abdominal pain. Mrs. Stevens had mild, crampy vaginal bleeding associated with abdominal pain. The most likely diagnosis in this patient is a threatened abortion. Pelvic examination reveals a closed cervical os and ultrasonography should demonstrate a viable fetus in this patient.

Mr. and Mrs. Stevens will be informed of the diagnosis. The chances of carrying the pregnancy to term are good. Restricting coitus and exercise for several weeks after bleeding has stopped is advised. The physician should offer support and reassurance to these anxious future parents.

Patient Note Pearl: The **differential diagnosis** for this patient includes threatened abortion, incomplete abortion, complete abortion, postcoital bleeding, ectopic pregnancy, and trophoblastic disease. The **diagnostic workup** includes a pelvic examination, CBC, pelvic sonography, and a pregnancy test.

Case 38

A 30-year-old investment banker, Victoria Billingsley, has made an appointment to see you for her annual gynecologic examination. Her regular gynecologist retired to Florida, and she is seeing you for the first time.

She wants to be evaluated for worsening menstrual cramps. The nurse practitioner informs you that the gynecologic examination is positive for a tender, fixed, retroverted uterus, indurated nodules in the cul-de-sac, left ovary enlargement and no adnexal or cervical motion tenderness.

Vital Signs:

Temperature	98.6°F
Blood pressure	115/75 mmHg
Heart rate	80 beats per minute
Respiratory rate	12 breaths per minute

Examinee's Tasks
(Do not repeat gynecologic examination)

1. Obtain a focused and relevant history.

2. Discuss your initial diagnostic impressions with the patient.

3. Discuss follow-up tests with the patient.

4. Provide patient education.

5. After seeing the patient, complete paperwork relevant to the case.

MY CHECKLIST

History of Present Illness. The Examinee:

1. _____
2. _____
3. _____
   _____
4. _____
5. _____
6. _____
7. _____
8. _____
   _____
   _____
9. _____
10. _____
11. _____
12. _____

Communication Skills. The Examinee:

13. _____
14. _____
15. _____
16. _____
17. _____
18. _____
19. _____

SP CHECKLIST FOR MS. BILLINGSLEY

History of Present Illness. The Examinee:

___ 1. asked about the onset of the worsening menstrual cramps ("The last 10 months have been terrible.")

___ 2. asked about the severity of the cramps ("I have to miss work 2 days every month.")

___ 3. asked about any alleviating factors ("At this point, bed rest is all that works; I've tried over-the-counter medications and none of them work.")

___ 4. asked about any changes in the amount of menstrual flow ("The amount seems to be the same.")

___ 5. asked about my last menstrual period ("It was 8 days ago and I missed 3 days of work.")

___ 6. asked about my last Pap smear ("13 months ago and it was normal.")

___ 7. asked about my obstetric history ("No history of pregnancies.")

___ 8. asked about previous attempts at pregnancy ("I was married for 5 years and used no contraception; I never became pregnant. My husband and I were not serious about having children at the time, so we didn't seek help. I always thought I might be infertile.")

___ 9. asked about a history of any gynecologic problems, i.e., endometriosis or sexually transmitted diseases ("Never.")

___10. asked about a family history of gynecologic problems, e.g., endometriosis ("None.")

___11. asked about any dyspareunia ("Yes.")

___12. asked about my sexual history ("One partner for 2 years; monogamous; no method of contraception.")

Communication Skills. The Examinee:

___13. explained the diagnostic possibilities to me (i.e., endometriosis, adhesions, myoma).

___14. explained what was needed to confirm the diagnosis (laparoscopy).

___15. explained the complications of these problems (infertility, chronic pain).

___16. explained the importance of follow-up for the problem.

___17. offered to give me ongoing support.

___18. asked me if I had any other questions or concerns.

___19. reassured me that infertility can often be corrected.

If you performed 14 of these 19 tasks, you passed this test station.

You have 10 minutes to complete your patient note.

HISTORY—Include significant positives and negatives from the history of present illness, past medical history, review of systems, and social and family history.

_____
_____
_____
_____
_____
_____
_____
_____
_____
_____

PHYSICAL EXAMINATION—Indicate only the pertinent positive and negative findings related to the patient's chief complaint.

_____
_____
_____
_____
_____
_____
_____
_____
_____
_____

DIFFERENTIAL DIAGNOSIS—In order of likelihood, write no more than five differential diagnoses for this patient's current problems.

1. _____
2. _____
3. _____
4. _____
5. _____

DIAGNOSTIC WORKUP—Immediate plans for no more than five diagnostic studies.

1. _____
2. _____
3. _____
4. _____
5. _____

A SATISFACTORY PATIENT NOTE

HISTORY—Include significant positives and negatives from the history of present illness, past medical history, review of systems, and social and family history.

Ms. Victoria Billingsley, 30 years old, has a 10-month history of painful menses. The cramps are so painful that she has had to miss 2 days of work every month. Her LMP was 8 days ago and the pain caused her to miss 3 days of work. Her menstrual flow is normal. Bed rest alleviates the pain, but over-the-counter medications are not helpful. She has never been pregnant and her Pap smear 13 months ago was normal. She was married for 5 years, used no contraception, and never became pregnant. She thought at the time that either she or her husband was infertile. She has no history of sexually transmitted disease and has never been diagnosed with endometriosis. She has no family history of gynecologic disease. She is monogamous with one sexual partner and uses no contraception. She has dyspareunia.

PHYSICAL EXAMINATION—Indicate only the pertinent positive and negative findings related to the patient's chief complaint.

Gynecologic: Tender, fixed, retroverted uterus, indurated nodules in the cul-de-sac, left ovary enlargement and no adnexal or cervical motion tenderness.

DIFFERENTIAL DIAGNOSIS
In order of likelihood, write no more than five differential diagnoses for this patient's current problems.

1. dysmenorrhea
2. endometriosis
3. adhesions
4. myoma
5.

DIAGNOSTIC WORKUP
Immediate plans for no more than five diagnostic studies.

1. pelvic ultrasound
2. laparoscopy
3.
4.
5.

LEARNING OBJECTIVE FOR MS. BILLINGSLEY
RECOGNIZE AND EVALUATE INFERTILITY

Ms. Billingsley presents with the chief complaint of worsening menstrual cramps without changes in menstrual flow. She also complains of dyspareunia. She has no history of previous pregnancies or gynecologic problems. Her history is suspicious for infertility (5-year marriage with no contraception use).

Women with endometriosis present with a chief complaint of infertility or worsening menstrual cramps. Dyspareunia may also be the presenting problem. Often, there is a family history of endometriosis.

Detection of nodules (endometriomas) or an adnexal mass on pelvic examination is usually found in advanced cases of endometriosis. The physical examination in early or minimal disease may be normal. Ms. Billingsley will need laparoscopy for definitive diagnosis and to document the extent and stage of her disease. She will be counseled regarding the benefits of surgical intervention (remove endometriomas and lyse adhesions) to correct infertility and to alleviate the symptoms of endometriosis.

Patient Note Pearl: The **differential diagnosis** for infertility (failure to conceive after 1 year of intercourse without contraception) includes the male factor (endocrine abnormalities such as hypopituitarism, drug- or tumor-induced hyperprolactinemia, thyroid and adrenal dysfunction), abnormal spermatogenesis (orchitis), anatomic problems, motility problems, and sexual dysfunction (impotence, retrograde ejaculation). The female factor may include problems with central ovulation (hyperprolactinemia, hypopituitarism), peripheral ovulation (ovarian resistance, premature ovarian failure), pelvic problems [endometriosis, adhesions, diethylstilbestrol (DES) exposure, myoma, PID], and cervical problems (DES). The **initial diagnostic workup** is based on the history of both partners and the pelvic examination but may include semen analysis, luteinizing hormone (LH), follicle-stimulating hormone (FSH), and prolactin levels.

Case 39

Mrs. Mary Michaels, 25 years old, presents to your office for a prenatal visit. She recently moved to your town and heard from her landlady that you were an excellent physician.

Vital Signs:

Temperature	98.6°F
Blood pressure	110/80 mmHg
Heart rate	86 beats per minute
Respiratory rate	12 breaths per minute

Examinee's Tasks

1. Obtain a focused and relevant history.

2. Discuss your initial diagnostic impressions with the patient.

3. Discuss follow-up tests with the patient.

4. Provide patient education.

5. After seeing the patient, complete paperwork relevant to the case.

MY CHECKLIST

History of Present Illness. The Examinee:

1. _____
2. _____
   _____
3. _____
4. _____
   _____
   _____
5. _____
6. _____
7. _____
8. _____
9. _____
10. _____
11. _____
12. _____
13. _____
    _____
14. _____

Communication Skills. The Examinee:

15. _____
16. _____
17. _____
    _____
18. _____
19. _____
20. _____
21. _____
22. _____
23. _____
24. _____
25. _____
26. _____

SP CHECKLIST FOR MRS. MICHAELS

History of Present Illness. The Examinee:

___ 1. asked about my last menstrual period ("I'm not exactly sure. I think around 5 months ago.")

___ 2. asked about my obstetric history ("This is my second attempt for a baby; I had a miscarriage 3 years ago in my fifth week.")

___ 3. asked about a history of sexually transmitted disease, i.e., herpes, gonorrhea, *Chlamydia*, syphilis, HIV ("No.")

___ 4. asked about my other ob/gyn history, i.e., menarche, regular periods, contraception, prior gyn surgery ("Menarche at 13 years old, regular periods, no contraception, monogamous with husband, no gyn surgery in the past.")

___ 5. asked about any pregnancy-related complaints, i.e., abdominal pain, vaginal bleeding ("No.")

___ 6. asked about a history of medical problems ("None.")

___ 7. asked about a history of previous blood transfusions ("No.")

___ 8. asked about any prenatal care ("None. We could not afford it before, but now my husband has a job.")

___ 9. asked about any tobacco use ("No.")

___10. asked about any alcohol use ("None.")

___11. asked about any illicit drug use ("None.")

___12. asked about my diet ("I try to eat three well-balanced meals a day.")

___13. asked about a history of congenital or birth problems in my family or my husband's family, i.e., cerebral palsy or Down's syndrome ("No.")

___14. asked if I felt fetal movements ("Oh, yes. I started feeling them just a couple of days ago.")

Communication Skills. The Examinee:

___15. asked about support from my husband ("Yes. He is very much involved.")

___16. told me I would receive help from a nutritionist for optimal diet instruction.

___17. explained that I would need blood drawn to check for previous infections, i.e., hepatitis, rubella, syphilis, and HIV (I must consent to HIV testing).

___18. explained that I would need blood drawn to check for anemia, i.e., low blood count.

___19. explained that I would need a sonogram to check the baby.

___20. explained that I would need a Pap smear done.

___21. explained that I would need to give a urine sample to check for a urinary tract infection without symptoms.

___22. explained that I would need to come to the doctor on a regular basis.

___23. explained the need for vitamins with iron for the baby.

___24. discussed community resources that prepare parents for labor and delivery.

___25. asked about a couples' appointment next time so my husband could participate.

___26. solicited questions from me.

If you performed 19 of these 26 tasks, you passed this test station.

You have 10 minutes to complete your patient note.

HISTORY—Include significant positives and negatives from the history of present illness, past medical history, review of systems, and social and family history.

_____
_____
_____
_____
_____
_____
_____
_____
_____
_____
_____

PHYSICAL EXAMINATION—Indicate only the pertinent positive and negative findings related to the patient's chief complaint.

_____
_____
_____
_____
_____
_____
_____
_____
_____
_____
_____

DIFFERENTIAL DIAGNOSIS—In order of likelihood, write no more than five differential diagnoses for this patient's current problems.

1. _____
2. _____
3. _____
4. _____
5. _____

DIAGNOSTIC WORKUP—Immediate plans for no more than five diagnostic studies.

1. _____
2. _____
3. _____
4. _____
5. _____

A SATISFACTORY PATIENT NOTE

HISTORY—Include significant positives and negatives from the history of present illness, past medical history, review of systems, and social and family history.

Mrs. Mary Michaels is a 25-year-old woman who presents for her first prenatal visit. She is G2P0 and her LMP was 5 months ago. She was 13 years old at the time of menarche and has always had regular periods. She has no history of sexually transmitted diseases and has no prior gynecologic history. She had a miscarriage 3 years ago in her first trimester. She is monogamous with her husband of 4 years and does not use any contraception. She has no history of medical problems, such as diabetes, asthma or, hypertension, and has never required a blood transfusion. She wanted to come for prenatal care sooner but her husband was unemployed until recently. She confirmed her pregnancy with a home pregnancy kit 3 months ago. She has no complaints and denies abdominal pain and vaginal bleeding. She does not smoke cigarettes, drink alcohol, or use illicit drugs. She tries to eat three well-balanced meals per day. She has no history of congenital or birth problems in her or her husband's family. She started to feel fetal movements just a few days ago. She is unsure as to how much weight she has gained since becoming pregnant.

PHYSICAL EXAMINATION—Indicate only the pertinent positive and negative findings related to the patient's chief complaint.

Temperature	98.6°F
Blood pressure	110/80 mmHg
Heart rate	86 beats per minute
Respiratory rate	12 breaths per minute

The patient, a pleasant and friendly young woman, is in her fifth month of pregnancy and in NAD.

DIFFERENTIAL DIAGNOSIS
In order of likelihood, write no more than five differential diagnoses for this patient's current problems.

1. pregnancy
2. lack of prenatal care
3.
4.
5.

DIAGNOSTIC WORKUP
Immediate plans for no more than five diagnostic studies.

1. pregnancy test
2. pelvic sonogram
3. serology for HIV, hepatitis, rubella, and syphilis
4. CBC
5. urine culture

LEARNING OBJECTIVE FOR MRS. MICHAELS
APPROPRIATE PRENATAL COUNSELING

Mrs. Michaels presents to your office for her first prenatal visit. She denies using any substances that are harmful to the fetus, including illicit drugs, alcohol, and tobacco. She has no past history of medical problems such as hypertension, diabetes, or asthma. She has no prior history of sexually transmitted diseases that might complicate delivery. Neither parent-to-be has any family history of cerebral palsy, Down's syndrome, or multiple births.

During the first trimester, laboratory studies should include blood type with antibody screen, hepatitis B serology, *Treponema* antibody, and rubella titers. An HIV test should be obtained with informed consent. A CBC is necessary to check for anemia and thrombocytopenia. Hemoglobin electrophoresis is necessary when indicated by the history. A physician should perform a Pap test and screen for gonorrhea and *Chlamydia*. Urine culture should be sent to detect asymptomatic bacteriuria.

The patient should be counseled regarding diet and weight gain (no more than 30 pounds during the pregnancy) and made aware that moderate exercise and sexual intercourse are safe during pregnancy.

During the second trimester, the patient is offered testing for the serum maternal α-fetoprotein (SMAFP) level (for detection of neural tube defects) and trisomies. Older women or high-risk patients require genetic counseling. Fetal movements should be felt by the patient around the 16th week of pregnancy (possibly not until the 20th week if the patient is primiparous). The third trimester requires screening for gestational diabetes mellitus.

Routine ultrasound examination of every pregnant patient is not necessary but will be done on Mrs. Michaels since she has no previous prenatal care (late registrant).

Education and counseling is an integral part of following a pregnant patient. The father should be involved in visits and discussions regarding all aspects of the pregnancy, including breast-feeding, labor, and delivery.

Patient Note Pearl: The **differential diagnosis** is second-trimester pregnancy and lack of prenatal care. The **diagnostic workup** includes pregnancy test, pelvic ultrasonography, blood type with antibody screen, hepatitis B serology, *Treponema* antibody, rubella titers, HIV test, CBC, urine culture, Pap test and screen for gonorrhea and *Chlamydia*.

Case 40

Mrs. Polly Peterson is a 37-year-old woman (AOG 30 weeks) G4P2 who presents to the emergency room with the complaint of vaginal bleeding.

Vital Signs:

Temperature	98.5°F
Blood pressure	130/70 mmHg
Heart rate	80 beats per minute
Respiratory rate	18 breaths per minute

Examinee's Tasks

1. Obtain a focused and relevant history.
2. Discuss your initial diagnostic impressions with the patient.
3. Discuss follow-up tests with the patient.
4. Provide patient education.
5. After seeing the patient, complete paperwork relevant to the case.

MY CHECKLIST

History of Present Illness. The Examinee:

1. _____
2. _____
3. _____
4. _____
5. _____
6. _____
   _____
7. _____
8. _____
9. _____
10. _____
11. _____
12. _____

Communication Skills. The Examinee:

13. _____
14. _____
15. _____
16. _____
17. _____
    _____
18. _____

SP CHECKLIST FOR MRS. PETERSON

History of Present Illness. The Examinee:

___ 1. asked about the onset of vaginal bleeding ("I woke up and found my bed soaked with bright red clotted blood.")

___ 2. asked about any associated pain ("I felt no pain but I did have some abdominal cramps.")

___ 3. asked about the quantity of blood loss ("It was very profuse but it has stopped now.")

___ 4. asked about a history of previous bleeding ("Some spotting during my fourth month.")

___ 5. asked about any problems in the course of this pregnancy ("No.")

___ 6. asked about the nature of the previous deliveries ("First child NSVD and second child by cesarean section; one spontaneous abortion.")

___ 7. asked about previous surgical procedures ("None.")

___ 8. asked about tobacco use ("None.")

___ 9. asked about alcohol use ("None.")

___10. asked about illicit drug use ("No.")

___11. asked about other medical problems ("None.")

___12. asked about fever or chills ("None.")

Communication Skills. The Examinee:

___13. seemed concerned about my anxiety.

___14. explained the most likely diagnosis (placenta previa or abruptio placentae).

___15. explained the rationale behind not performing gynecologic examination.

___16. explained the need for a sonogram to make a definitive diagnosis.

___17. explained that blood tests were needed to check clotting factors (CBC, PT, PTT, fibrinogen, fibrin split products).

___18. explained the plan (admission to the hospital, strict bed rest, fetal monitoring, and possible blood transfusions).

If you performed 13 of these 18 tasks, you passed this test station.

You have 10 minutes to complete your patient note.

HISTORY—Include significant positives and negatives from the history of present illness, past medical history, review of systems, and social and family history.

_____
_____
_____
_____
_____
_____
_____
_____
_____
_____

PHYSICAL EXAMINATION—Indicate only the pertinent positive and negative findings related to the patient's chief complaint.

_____
_____
_____
_____
_____
_____
_____
_____
_____
_____

DIFFERENTIAL DIAGNOSIS—In order of likelihood, write no more than five differential diagnoses for this patient's current problems.

1. _____
2. _____
3. _____
4. _____
5. _____

DIAGNOSTIC WORKUP—Immediate plans for no more than five diagnostic studies.

1. _____
2. _____
3. _____
4. _____
5. _____

A SATISFACTORY PATIENT NOTE

HISTORY—Include significant positives and negatives from the history of present illness, past medical history, review of systems, and social and family history.

Mrs. Polly Peterson, 37 years old, is a G4P2 with an AOG of 30 weeks. When she awoke this morning she found her bed soaked with blood clots due to profuse vaginal bleeding. The bleeding has now stopped. She had some mild abdominal cramps but no abdominal pain. She denies fever and chills. Her only problem during pregnancy has been some spotting in her fourth month, but her obstetrician told her that is was normal and not dangerous. Aside from the spotting, she had no other pregnancy problems. Her obstetric history is positive for a child born by cesarean section, another child was a NSVD, and one spontaneous abortion. She has been compliant with her prenatal appointments and diet. She does not smoke cigarettes, drink alcohol, or use illicit drugs. She has no previous surgical history and no medical problems.

PHYSICAL EXAMINATION—Indicate only the pertinent positive and negative findings related to the patient's chief complaint.

T = 98.5. BP = 130/70 mmHg. HR = 80 beats/min. RR = 18 breaths/min.
A frightened and anxious 37-year-old woman AOG 30 weeks. She is tearful and appears to be very concerned.

DIFFERENTIAL DIAGNOSIS
In order of likelihood, write no more than five differential diagnoses for this patient's current problems.

1. placenta previa
2. abruptio placenta
3. cervical dilatation
4. coagulation disorder
5. vaginal lesion

DIAGNOSTIC WORKUP
Immediate plans for no more than five diagnostic studies.

1. CBC
2. PT and PTT
3. transabdominal ultrasound
4.
5.

LEARNING OBJECTIVE FOR MRS. PETERSON
APPROACH TO THE PATIENT WITH THIRD-TRIMESTER BLEEDING

The most common causes of life-threatening third-trimester bleeding are placenta previa (implantation of the placenta over or near the internal os) and abruptio placentae (premature separation of a normally implanted placenta prior to fetal delivery). Less severe third-trimester bleeding may be secondary to extrauterine sources, such as cervical trauma, cervical dilatation, coagulation disorders, and vaginal or rectal lesions.

Mrs. Peterson is at increased risk for placenta previa given her advanced maternal age, multiparity, and prior C-section. Predisposing factors for abruptio placentae include advanced maternal age, multiparity, diabetes, hypertension, prior abruption, smoking, alcohol use, and cocaine use.

Painless vaginal bleeding is the cardinal sign of placenta previa and differentiates it from abruptio placentae, which may present with unremitting abdominal (uterine) low back pain.

Hemorrhage may be visible or concealed. There may also be evidence of fetal distress, disseminated intravascular coagulation, or hypovolemic shock.

Transabdominal ultrasonography demonstrates the placement and separation of the placenta and includes assessment of fetal well-being, gestational age, and localization of amniotic fluid.

For minor bleeding, bed rest is recommended. If uterine contractions are present, tocolytics can be used. For severe bleeding, the patient must be stabilized and delivered by C-section. Subsequent management is dictated by maternal stability (bleeding may be unpredictable and persistent), fetal stability, and gestational age.

Physical Examination Pearl: A vaginal or rectal examination should NOT be done until placenta previa has been ruled out. The most gentle pelvic examination may provoke an uncontrollable hemorrhage.

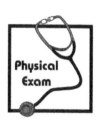

Patient Note Pearl: The **differential diagnosis** for third-trimester bleeding includes placenta previa, abruptio placentae, cervical trauma, cervical dilatation, coagulation disorders, and vaginal or rectal lesions. The **diagnostic workup** may include a CBC, PT, PTT, and transabdominal ultrasonography. A pelvic examination may be contraindicated in patients with placenta previa.

Case 41

Your patient is a 20-year-old woman named Linda Luckey. Her mother has scheduled this appointment because she feels her daughter is overly concerned with her weight. The mother is afraid that her daughter may have an eating disorder.

Upon entering the examination room, you see a cachectic-appearing young woman with thin, fine hair. She is approximately 5 feet 7 inches tall and weighs 105 pounds.

Vital Signs:

Temperature	96.0°F
Blood pressure	85/60 mmHg
Heart rate	48 beats per minute
Respirations	12 breaths per minute

Examinee's Tasks

1. Obtain a focused and relevant history.
2. Discuss your initial diagnostic impressions with the patient.
3. Discuss follow-up tests with the patient.
4. After seeing the patient, complete paperwork relevant to the case.

MY CHECKLIST

History of Present Illness. The Examinee:

1. _____
2. _____
3. _____
4. _____
5. _____
6. _____
7. _____
   _____
8. _____
9. _____
10. _____
11. _____
    _____
12. _____
13. _____
14. _____
15. _____
    _____

Communication Skills. The Examinee:

16. _____
17. _____
18. _____
19. _____
20. _____
21. _____
22. _____
23. _____

SP CHECKLIST FOR MS. LUCKEY

History of Present Illness. The Examinee:

___ 1. asked about my weight loss ("I don't feel like I'm losing weight; I'm not sure why Mom is so worried.")

___ 2. asked about my diet ("I eat lots of fruits and vegetables; I stay away from fatty foods and high carbs.")

___ 3. asked if I skip any meals ("Yes, sometimes breakfast or lunch; sometimes dinner. Fasting is healthy.")

___ 4. asked if I have secret food binges ("Yes, I have binge weekends.")

___ 5. asked about self-induced vomiting ("No.")

___ 6. asked about the use of laxatives or diuretics to help lose weight ("No.")

___ 7. asked if I count my caloric intake daily ("Yes, everyone should watch what they eat, shouldn't they? I try not to go above 1000 calories per day.")

___ 8. asked about ritualistic exercise ("I run 5 miles every day.")

___ 9. asked me if I felt fat ("Just my thighs and arms are fat; the rest of me is alright.")

___10. asked me if I had a fear of gaining weight ("Yes; I really don't want to be fat.")

___11. asked if I was preoccupied with my diet and food ("Well, I do think about food every day; I even collect recipes. I like to cook.")

___12. asked about my social life ("No time; I have to study.")

___13. asked about any sexual relationships ("None. I'm too busy.")

___14. asked about any signs of depression, i.e., insomnia, crying ("No.")

___15. asked about amenorrhea ("No menstrual flow for 3 months; I think it's the stress of school. I want to go to an Ivy League school and be a lawyer.")

Communication Skills. The Examinee:

___16. discussed the initial impression with me (i.e., eating disorder, major depression, thyroid disease).

___17. discussed the workup with me (blood work, thyroid tests, electrocardiogram).

___18. discussed why hospitalization was needed.

___19. discussed the fact that treatment would include behavioral therapy and medication.

___20. discussed the entire family's need to participate in my care (family counseling).

___21. discussed my need for nutritional support.

___22. inquired about my understanding of the problem.

___23. was supportive.

If you performed 17 of these 23 tasks, you passed this test station.

You have 10 minutes to complete your patient note.

HISTORY—Include significant positives and negatives from the history of present illness, past medical history, review of systems, and social and family history.

_____
_____
_____
_____
_____
_____
_____
_____
_____
_____

PHYSICAL EXAMINATION—Indicate only the pertinent positive and negative findings related to the patient's chief complaint.

_____
_____
_____
_____
_____
_____
_____
_____
_____
_____

DIFFERENTIAL DIAGNOSIS—In order of likelihood, write no more than five differential diagnoses for this patient's current problems.

1. _____
2. _____
3. _____
4. _____
5. _____

DIAGNOSTIC WORKUP—Immediate plans for no more than five diagnostic studies.

1. _____
2. _____
3. _____
4. _____
5. _____

A SATISFACTORY PATIENT NOTE

HISTORY—Include significant positives and negatives from the history of present illness, past medical history, review of systems, and social and family history.

Twenty-year-old Ms. Linda Luckey is brought to your office by her mother for evaluation of weight loss. The patient does not feel that she has lost any weight and is unsure why her mother has scheduled the appointment. Ms. Luckey's diet consists mainly of fruits and vegetables; she stays away from foods high in fats and carbohydrates. She sometimes fasts and often skips meals. She has secret food binges on weekends but denies inducing vomiting or using laxatives or diuretics in an attempt to lose weight. She counts her daily calories and tries not to go above 1000 calories per day and often runs 5 miles a day to stay in shape. She is preoccupied with food and diet; she collects recipes and likes to cook. Her self-image is such that she feels that her thighs and arms are fat; she has a fear of gaining any more weight. She has few friends and no sexual relationships because she is too busy studying to get into an Ivy League law school. Her last menstrual period was 3 months ago and she feels that the stress of school has made her periods irregular. She does not think she is depressed and denies insomnia, sadness, or episodes of crying.

PHYSICAL EXAMINATION—Indicate only the pertinent positive and negative findings related to the patient's chief complaint.

The patient is a cachectic-appearing young woman with thin, fine hair. She is approximately 5 feet 7 inches tall and weighs 105 pounds. She looks older than her stated age of 20 years. She is hypothermic, hypotensive, and bradycardic.

DIFFERENTIAL DIAGNOSIS
In order of likelihood, write no more than five differential diagnoses for this patient's current problems.

1. anorexia nervosa
2. hypothyroidism
3. major depression
4. hypothermia
5. bradycardia

DIAGNOSTIC WORKUP
Immediate plans for no more than five diagnostic studies.

1. CBC
2. electrolytes
3. BUN and creatinine
4. TSH
5. ECG

LEARNING OBJECTIVE FOR MS. LUCKEY
APPROACH TO THE YOUNG WOMAN WITH WEIGHT LOSS

Ms. Linda Luckey is a 20-year-old college student who wishes to become an attorney. Her dream is to attend an Ivy League law school and be a corporate lawyer like her parents. She is described by family and friends as a goal-oriented perfectionist driven by her desire for success and achievement. She has little time for social relationships and is focused on performing well in school.

This cachectic young woman weighs 105 pounds, which is less than 85 percent of her expected body weight. She limits her daily caloric intake and avoids foods high in fats and carbohydrates. She secretly binges on food on weekends but denies self-induced vomiting or the use of laxatives and diuretics in an attempt to lose weight. She tries to remain thin by fasting and exercising to excess. She has a distorted image of her underweight body and considers specific areas (thighs and arms) to be fat. Recently, she has become amenorrheic. All the information obtained in the history is consistent with the diagnosis of anorexia nervosa.

Anorexia nervosa is 20 times more common in women than in men. A patient will present after having lost a significant percentage of his or her expected body weight and will typically be preoccupied with food, body weight, and daily caloric intake.

Ms. Luckey feels herself to be a healthy, average young woman and denies her symptoms (denial of the problem is frequently seen in eating disorders). Her parents, however, are concerned about anorexia nervosa and have coerced their daughter into seeking psychiatric help.

On presentation, the patient is hypothermic, bradycardic, and hypotensive. Her hair is fine and thin (lanugo). This presentation is consistent with severe malnutrition secondary to anorexia nervosa.

The treatment of anorexia nervosa includes family counseling, nutritional support, medication use, and hospitalization. Ms. Luckey will need these interventions to achieve and maintain an adequate weight. Death in patients with anorexia nervosa may occur secondary to cardiac arrhythmias, electrolyte abnormalities, or suicide.

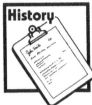

History-Taking Pearl: Try to differentiate between anorexia nervosa and bulimia by history:

	anorexia nervosa	bulimia
weight control methods	decreased intake	self-induced vomiting and laxative use
weight	markedly decreased	may be near normal
binge eating	uncommon	common
ritualized exercise	common	rare
hypotension and bradycardia	common	uncommon
medical complications	hypokalemia and arrhythmias	hypokalemia, arrhythmias, and esophageal rupture

Patient Note Pearl: Before making the diagnosis of anorexia nervosa, medical conditions such as thyroid disease, diabetes mellitus, malignancy, and HIV must be excluded. The **differential diagnosis** of an eating disorder includes major depression and obsessive-compulsive disorder.

NOTES

Case 42

Michael Minty, a 45-year-old architect, has made an appointment to see you at the suggestion of his two sisters. The Minty sisters feel that Michael is despondent over the sudden death of his wife in a motor vehicle accident. They had been married less than a year at the time. The sisters are afraid that their brother will commit suicide. You are the psychiatrist evaluating Mr. Minty.

Vital Signs:

Temperature	98.6°F
Blood pressure	125/80 mmHg
Heart rate	84 beats per minute
Respiratory rate	12 breaths per minute

Examinee's Tasks

1. Obtain a focused and relevant history.

2. Discuss your initial diagnostic impressions with the patient.

3. Discuss follow-up tests with the patient.

4. After seeing the patient, complete paperwork relevant to the case.

MY CHECKLIST

History of Present Illness. The Examinee:

1. _____
2. _____
_____
3. _____
_____
4. _____
5. _____
6. _____
7. _____
_____
8. _____
_____
9. _____
10. _____
11. _____
12. _____
_____

Communication Skills. The Examinee:

13. _____
14. _____
15. _____
16. _____
17. _____
18. _____

SP CHECKLIST FOR MR. MINTY

History of Present Illness. The Examinee:

___ 1. asked how long ago my wife died ("4 months ago.")

___ 2. asked if I was angry about my wife dying ("Yes; I'm very angry about it. I'm also sad and lonely. It took me 25 years to find the right woman to marry.")

___ 3. asked if I felt guilty about my wife's death ("Yes; she died a horrible death. I should have taken her to the store that night; it was raining.")

___ 4. asked if I had problems sleeping ("Yes; I sleep only 4 hours every night.")

___ 5. asked if I have any dreams about my wife ("Yes; I dream about her all the time.")

___ 6. asked about any loss of appetite ("Yes; I just don't feel like eating. I sometimes skip meals.")

___ 7. asked what I do in my free time ("I work on my wife's stamp collection; she would have liked that. I don't leave the house very much.")

___ 8. asked about withdrawing from the family ("I just need to be alone for a while, that's all. Sometimes I need to cry a little.")

___ 9. asked me about any new relationships ("I'm not ready to date or initiate a relationship right now.")

___10. asked me about my work ("I was just promoted at work; everything at work is great.")

___11. asked about any alcohol use ("No.")

___12. asked about any drug use ("Absolutely not; a friend of mine gave me some sleeping pills but I refuse to take them; I dislike medications.")

Communication Skills. The Examinee:

___13. discussed the impression with me (normal grief reaction).

___14. explained that I will feel like participating in life again eventually.

___15. explained that the grief will recede eventually.

___16. explained to me that everything I am feeling is perfectly normal.

___17. offered to speak to my sisters about the problem.

___18. offered ongoing support.

If you performed 13 of these 18 tasks, you passed this test station.

You have 10 minutes to complete your patient note.

HISTORY—Include significant positives and negatives from the history of present illness, past medical history, review of systems, and social and family history.

_____
_____
_____
_____
_____
_____
_____
_____
_____
_____
_____

PHYSICAL EXAMINATION—Indicate only the pertinent positive and negative findings related to the patient's chief complaint.

_____
_____
_____
_____
_____
_____
_____
_____
_____
_____
_____

DIFFERENTIAL DIAGNOSIS—In order of likelihood, write no more than five differential diagnoses for this patient's current problems.

1. _____
2. _____
3. _____
4. _____
5. _____

DIAGNOSTIC WORKUP—Immediate plans for no more than five diagnostic studies.

1. _____
2. _____
3. _____
4. _____
5. _____

A SATISFACTORY PATIENT NOTE

HISTORY—Include significant positives and negatives from the history of present illness, past medical history, review of systems, and social and family history.

Mr. Michael Minty is a 45-year-old architect who for 4 months has been grieving the death of his wife of less than a year, who died in a motor vehicle accident. This occurred on a rainy night and Mr. Minty is feeling guilty that he let his wife drive and did not drive her to the store. He is angry and upset that she died such a horrible death and holds himself responsible. Since her death, he is sleeping only 4 hours a night, and his dreams revolve around his wife. He has no appetite and often skips meals. He occasionally cries and feels sad and lonely. He feels that he needs to spend some time by himself and has withdrawn from members of the family. He doesn't leave the house very often and spends his free time working on his wife's stamp collection. Although his sisters want Mr. Minty to start dating other women, he feels that he is not ready to initiate a relationship. He is a successful architect and was recently promoted. He does not use alcohol and he takes no medications.

PHYSICAL EXAMINATION—Indicate only the pertinent positive and negative findings related to the patient's chief complaint.

T = 98.6°F. BP = 125/80 mmHg. HR = 84 beats/min. RR = 12 breaths/min.
The patient is a well-developed, well-nourished male who is in NAD. He is pleasant and cooperative; not tearful or anxious.

DIFFERENTIAL DIAGNOSIS
In order of likelihood, write no more than 5 differential diagnoses for this patient's current problems.

1. grief reaction
2. depression
3.
4.
5.

DIAGNOSTIC WORKUP
Immediate plans for no more than five diagnostic studies.

1. support only
2.
3.
4.
5.

LEARNING OBJECTIVE FOR MR. MINTY
DIFFERENTIATE BETWEEN NORMAL GRIEF AND DEPRESSION

Mr. Minty is experiencing a normal grief reaction. Since his wife's sudden death 4 months ago, he has had difficulty sleeping and has lost his appetite. When he does sleep, he dreams of his wife (which is part of normal grieving) and the good times they shared. He sometimes cries and admits to feeling sad and lonely. He rarely leaves the house to visit relatives and has no desire to establish new relationships.

The patient feels guilty and angry about the death of his wife. He has taken on some of her hobbies in an effort to feel closer to her. Everything else in his life is stable. He was recently promoted at his job. He has not used drugs or alcohol since his wife's death. He has withdrawn socially and does not want a new relationship at this time, but that is a normal part of grieving.

Mr. Minty's sisters are anxious and concerned about their brother. The patient's grief, however, is normal. Medications are not indicated. Mr. Minty must simply undergo the mourning process. As grief recedes, the patient will begin to participate in old and new relationships.

History-Taking Pearl: A grief reaction becomes abnormal when the patient develops extreme vegetative symptoms such as a profoundly depressed mood and a major sleep disturbance. The patient will feel worthless and hopeless and will have active thoughts of suicide. Remember that the 6 to 12 months often quoted as the time frame for normal grieving may not apply to every situation.

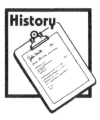

Patient Note Pearl: The **differential diagnosis** is grief reaction and depression. The **diagnostic workup** includes support and perhaps counseling.

Case 43

A 26-year-old woman, Tammy Tulip, has made an appointment to see you at the suggestion of her primary care physician. She has seen her private doctor eight times in the last 2 months for chest pain and has had an extensive workup including blood work (normal, including the lipid profile), an echocardiogram (normal), cardiac stress test (normal) and gastrointestinal studies (no esophageal spasm, GERD, or hiatal hernia).

Her private physician feels that Ms. Tulip must learn to relax and suggested your name for help and guidance. She continues to have frequent chest pain.

Vital Signs:

Temperature	98.7°F
Blood pressure	110/70 mmHg
Heart rate	76 beats per minute
Respiratory rate	12 breaths per minute

Examinee's Tasks

1. Obtain a focused and relevant history.
2. Obtain a focused and relevant physical examination.
3. Discuss your initial diagnostic impressions with the patient.
4. Discuss follow-up tests with the patient.
5. Provide patient education.
6. After seeing the patient, complete paperwork relevant to the case.

MY CHECKLIST

History of Present Illness. The Examinee:

1. _____
2. _____
3. _____
4. _____
5. _____
   _____
6. _____
7. _____
   _____
8. _____
   _____
9. _____
   _____
10. _____
    _____
11. _____
12. _____
13. _____
14. _____
15. _____

Physical Examination. The Examinee:

16. _____
17. _____
18. _____

Communication Skills. The Examinee:

19. _____
20. _____
21. _____
22. _____
23. _____
24. _____
25. _____

SP CHECKLIST FOR MS. TULIP

History of Present Illness. The Examinee:

___ 1. asked about the onset of the chest pain ("It started maybe a year ago.")

___ 2. asked about quality of chest pain ("Very sharp and worse if I move around.")

___ 2. asked about the location of the chest pain ("Middle of my chest.")

___ 3. asked about the frequency of the chest pain ("Maybe three episodes per week.")

___ 4. asked about the duration of each chest pain episode ("It lasts 15 minutes.")

___ 5. asked what precipitates the chest pain ("It's unpredictable; I may be in the movies, eating dinner, or driving the car; it can happen anytime.")

___ 6. asked about any alleviating factors ("I just try to relax, breathe slow, and it goes away on its own.")

___ 7. asked about any associated symptoms, i.e., dizziness, palpitations, diaphoresis, paresthesias, trembling, hyperventilating, suffocation ("Yes; I get all of those things.")

___ 8. asked about a fear of dying or a sense of terror with the chest pain ("Yes. That's why I call 911 when it happens.")

___ 9. asked if I was limiting or avoiding activities because of the chest pain ("I stopped going to the movies or to a restaurant because I'm afraid I may get an attack there.")

___10. asked about any family stresses, e.g., recent family death, family illness, marital problems ("None. I'm not married. I live alone. No children either.")

___11. asked about any job stresses ("I work as a toll collector; no stress whatsoever. I love my job.")

___12. asked if I experienced any trauma in my life, e.g., sexual abuse, child abuse, assault ("No, thank goodness.")

___12. asked about any tobacco abuse ("No.")

___13. asked about any alcohol use ("One glass of wine every night. I heard it's good for the heart.")

___14. asked about any illicit drug use ("No.")

___15. asked about any medication use ("My doctor gave me some pills for my nerves, but I never use them.")

Physical Examination. The Examinee:

___16. checked my thyroid gland by palpation (normal thyroid gland).

___17. listened to my heart in four places (normal examination).

___18. Listened to my lungs (normal examination).

Communication Skills. The Examinee:

___19. explained the initial diagnostic possibilities to me (i.e., panic disorder, phobia, depression).

___20. explained that my problem was treatable.

___21. told me that my problem was an exaggeration of a normal fear.

___22. explained the treatment to me (behavioral therapy, possibly medications, psychotherapy).

___23. advised me not to avoid the places where the attacks take place.

___24. showed concern for my problem.

___25. offered me ongoing support.

If you performed 18 of these 25 tasks, you passed this test station.

You have 10 minutes to complete your patient note.

HISTORY—Include significant positives and negatives from the history of present illness, past medical history, review of systems, and social and family history.

_____
_____
_____
_____
_____
_____
_____
_____
_____
_____

PHYSICAL EXAMINATION—Indicate only the pertinent positive and negative findings related to the patient's chief complaint.

_____
_____
_____
_____
_____
_____
_____
_____
_____
_____

DIFFERENTIAL DIAGNOSIS—In order of likelihood, write no more than five differential diagnoses for this patient's current problems.

1. _____
2. _____
3. _____
4. _____
5. _____

DIAGNOSTIC WORKUP—Immediate plans for no more than five diagnostic studies.

1. _____
2. _____
3. _____
4. _____
5. _____

A SATISFACTORY PATIENT NOTE

HISTORY—Include significant positives and negatives from the history of present illness, past medical history, review of systems, and social and family history.

Ms. Tammy Tulip, 26 years old, has had a 2-month history of sharp chest pain. The pain is located in the middle of her chest and lasts about 15 minutes. She has approximately three chest pain episodes per week. The pain goes away on its own or with slow breathing and relaxation. There are associated palpitations, dizziness, diaphoresis, trembling, hyperventilating, paresthesias, and feelings of suffocation. Ms. Tulip has feelings of impending doom, terror, and dying while having these episodes and often calls 911. The pain is unpredictable and has occurred while she was at the movies, while eating dinner, and while driving her car. She often avoids going to a restaurant or the movies because she feels that she may have another attack there. She has no personal, family, or work problems that are causing her stress. She is happy in her job as a toll collector. She has never suffered any kind of trauma either as an adult or as a child. She does not smoke cigarettes or use illicit drugs. She drinks a glass of red wine every night because she heard it was good for her heart. She has a prescription for antianxiety medication but has not used it. She is single and has no children. She has seen her private physician eight times in the last 2 months and has had normal blood work, including lipid profile, echocardiogram, stress test, and gastrointestinal studies. The only advice her private physician gave her was to learn to relax. The patient is now seeking a second opinion.

PHYSICAL EXAMINATION—Indicate only the pertinent positive and negative findings related to the patient's chief complaint.

T = 98.7°F. BP = 110/70 mmHg. HR = 76 beats/min. RR = 12 breaths/min.
The patient is an anxious and concerned woman pacing throughout the examination room.
HEENT: Normal thyroid gland.
Lungs: Clear to auscultation.
Heart: S_1 and S_2 normal. No murmurs, rubs, or gallops.

DIFFERENTIAL DIAGNOSIS

In order of likelihood, write no more than five differential diagnoses for this patient's current problems.

1. panic disorder
2. hyperthyroidism
3. hyperventilation syndrome
4. depression
5. posttraumatic stress disorder

DIAGNOSTIC WORKUP

Immediate plans for no more than five diagnostic studies.

1. TSH level
2. support
3.
4.
5.

LEARNING OBJECTIVE FOR MS. TULIP
APPROACH TO THE "NERVOUS" PATIENT WITH MULTIPLE COMPLAINTS

Ms. Tulip has been to several physicians with the complaint of recurrent chest pain. She has no risk factors for cardiac disease, and an extensive cardiac and gastrointestinal evaluation was unremarkable. Her episodes of chest pain are unpredictable and are associated with palpitations, dizziness, diaphoresis, trembling, hyperventilation, and paresthesias.

The cardiac episodes are so intense that Ms. Tulip feels death is imminent with each attack. She called the paramedics on several occasions. The patient is so frightened that she tries to avoid any location or function where previous attacks have taken place.

Ms. Tulip denies feeling stressed about her family or job. She denies substance abuse. She has experienced no traumatic event in her life that may have caused posttraumatic stress disorder.

Ms. Tulip is suffering from panic disorder. The disorder may be preceded by a previous stressful life event. The patient must not continue to avoid the places where previous panic attacks have occurred (this may lead to agoraphobia). Treatment for this disorder includes behavioral therapy (relaxation, desensitization, controlled exposure) and cautious use of medications. Psychotherapy may help unveil the subconscious reason for the anxiety.

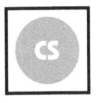

Patient Note Pearl: The **differential diagnosis** for panic disorder includes hyperthyroidism, hyperventilation syndrome, mitral valve prolapse, pheochromocytoma, SLE, vitamin B_{12} deficiency, and neurologic diseases including multiple sclerosis and Wilson's disease. Panic disorder symptoms should be differentiated from those of drug intoxication (cocaine, theophylline, amyl nitrite, amphetamines, anticholinergics) and drug withdrawal (alcohol, sedative hypnotics, antihypertensives). The **psychiatric differential diagnosis** for panic disorder includes hypochondriasis, malingering, depression, posttraumatic stress disorder (PTSD), simple phobia, and depersonalization. The **diagnostic workup** would include response to medication use, therapy, and counseling.

NOTES

Case 44

Eight weeks after having her first child, 32-year-old Mrs. Sadie Simmons (G1P1) makes an appointment to see you. Since the birth of her baby, Mrs. Simmons has been feeling emotionally drained.

Vital Signs:

Temperature	97.7°F
Blood pressure	105/70 mmHg
Heart rate	76 beats per minute
Respiratory rate	14 breaths per minute

Examinee's Tasks

1. Obtain a focused and relevant history.
2. Discuss your initial diagnostic impressions with the patient.
3. Discuss follow-up tests with the patient.
4. Provide patient education.
5. After seeing the patient, complete paperwork relevant to the case.

MY CHECKLIST

History of Present Illness. The Examinee:

1. _____
2. _____
   _____
3. _____
   _____
4. _____
   _____
5. _____
6. _____
7. _____
8. _____
   _____
9. _____
   _____
10. _____
11. _____
12. _____
13. _____
14. _____

Communication Skills. The Examinee:

15. _____
16. _____
17. _____
18. _____
19. _____
20. _____
21. _____
22. _____

SP CHECKLIST FOR MRS. SIMMONS

History of Present Illness. The Examinee:

___ 1. asked if my baby was healthy ("Yes.")

___ 2. asked if I was feeling anxious about caring for my baby ("Yes; this is all new to me; most of the time, I don't know if I'm doing it right.")

___ 3. asked about support from my husband ("He took on a second job to help with the bills; he is really tired when he comes home at night.")

___ 4. asked about communication difficulties with my husband ("I think he's stressed out about the baby; we don't talk as much as before.")

___ 5. asked if I felt less attractive to my husband ("Look at me; I gained so much weight.")

___ 6. asked about financial problems in the marriage ("We are just making ends meet.")

___ 7. asked about other family support systems ("My mother went home; she lives 1000 miles away.")

___ 8. asked me if I was feeling alone ("When the baby was first born, there were always visitors; now no one comes anymore.")

___ 9. asked me about mood changes, e.g., sleep disturbances, nightmares, loss of appetite, headache, fatigue, forgetfulness ("I am tired all the time; I have no energy.")

___10. asked if I ever thought about harming the baby ("Oh no, never.")

___11. asked about a history of psychiatric problems ("None.")

___12. asked me if I use tobacco ("I smoke 3 cigarettes a day.")

___13. asked me if I drink alcohol ("Maybe 2 beers a day.")

___14. asked me if I use illicit drugs ("No.")

Communication Skills. The Examinee:

___15. discussed the diagnosis with me [plausible diagnosis is postpartum depression (PPD)].

___16. explained the role of hormones in this problem.

___17. explained that the workup includes blood tests to check thyroid function.

___18. offered to speak to my husband and other family members to involve them in my care.

___19. offered me ongoing support.

___20. assessed my understanding of the problem.

___21. solicited my questions and concerns.

___22. scheduled a follow-up appointment.

If you performed 16 of these 22 tasks, you passed this test station.

You have 10 minutes to complete your patient note.

HISTORY—Include significant positives and negatives from the history of present illness, past medical history, review of systems, and social and family history.

_____

_____

_____

_____

_____

_____

_____

_____

_____

_____

PHYSICAL EXAMINATION—Indicate only the pertinent positive and negative findings related to the patient's chief complaint.

_____

_____

_____

_____

_____

_____

_____

_____

_____

_____

DIFFERENTIAL DIAGNOSIS—In order of likelihood, write no more than five differential diagnoses for this patient's current problems.

1. _____

2. _____

3. _____

4. _____

5. _____

DIAGNOSTIC WORKUP—Immediate plans for no more than five diagnostic studies.

1. _____

2. _____

3. _____

4. _____

5. _____

A SATISFACTORY PATIENT NOTE

HISTORY—Include significant positives and negatives from the history of present illness, past medical history, review of systems, and social and family history.

Mrs. Sadie Simmons, a 32-year-old woman (G1P1), is 8 weeks postpartum. Since the birth of her healthy baby, she has been feeling drained and has feelings of inadequacy regarding her ability to take care of the child. Her parents and other relatives were helpful during the pregnancy and shortly after she gave birth but have since returned to their homes far away. Now few people visit and there is little support. Her husband is rarely at home to help; he is working a second job for financial reasons and often comes home tired. Financially, the couple is just making ends meet. There is a breakdown in communication between them and she thinks that her husband might be feeling somewhat ignored and neglected since the baby was born. Additionally, because of her weight gain during pregnancy, she feels that her husband is probably finding her unattractive. Mrs. Simmons admits to feeling tired all the time and has no energy. She has no past history of psychiatric problems and has no thoughts of harming the baby. She smokes three cigarettes daily and drinks two beers; she does not use illicit drugs.

PHYSICAL EXAMINATION—Indicate only the pertinent positive and negative findings related to the patient's chief complaint.

T = 97.7°F. BP = 105/70 mmHg. HR = 76 beats/min. RR = 14 breaths/min.
The patient is a sad and tearful 32-year-old woman in NAD. She is slightly overweight.

DIFFERENTIAL DIAGNOSIS
In order of likelihood, write no more than five differential diagnoses for this patient's current problems.

1. postpartum depression
2. major depression
3.
4.
5.

DIAGNOSTIC WORKUP
Immediate plans for no more than five diagnostic studies.

1. support
2. medication
3. TSH level
4.
5.

LEARNING OBJECTIVE FOR MRS. SIMMONS
RECOGNIZE POSTPARTUM DEPRESSION

PPD may occur up to 1 year after the birth of a child. The new mother lacks confidence and will have feelings of inadequacy regarding her ability to take care of the newborn. Support systems that may have been helpful earlier during the pregnancy or shortly after giving birth (parents and relatives) may no longer be present in the household. The mother will be fatigued, irritable, anxious, and sleep-deprived. She may be tearful and sad. Occasionally, patients with PPD present with symptoms of psychosis.

The household changes that occur with a new baby may affect the relationship between husband and wife. The new mother may feel less attractive to her husband. The husband may feel ignored and neglected by the busy mother. Financial problems may further contribute to the problems. The situation may be worse if the newborn is ill or premature. The risk of postpartum mood disturbance is increased in women with prior episodes of major depressive disorder. The treatment of PPD includes improving the support system available to the new mother and enhancing communication between husband and wife. Medications are often required in the treatment of this disorder. There is an increased risk of infanticide with PPD, and the physician must screen for this throughout the treatment period.

History-Taking Pearl: It is essential for the physician to ask the mother about "ideas" regarding the infant. A depressed mother may be delusional and think the infant is ill and kill the infant to prevent it from suffering in the future.

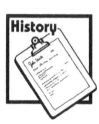

Patient Note Pearl: The **differential diagnosis** for postpartum depression includes major depressive disorder. The **diagnostic workup** may include a TSH level.

Case 45

Fifty-year-old Albert Sullivan presents to your office with the chief complaint of insomnia. He is requesting a prescription for sleeping pills. This is his first visit to your practice.

Vital Signs:

Temperature	98.7°F
Blood pressure	115/75 mmHg
Heart rate	80 beats per minute
Respiratory rate	12 breaths per minute

Examinee's Tasks

1. Obtain a focused and relevant history.
2. Discuss your initial diagnostic impressions with the patient.
3. Discuss follow-up tests with the patient.
4. Provide patient education.
5. After seeing the patient, complete paperwork relevant to the case.

MY CHECKLIST

History of Present Illness. The Examinee:

1. _____
2. _____
3. _____
4. _____
5. _____
   _____
6. _____
7. _____
   _____
8. _____
   _____
9. _____
10. _____
11. _____
    _____
12. _____
    _____
13. _____
14. _____
15. _____
16. _____
17. _____
18. _____

Communication Skills. The Examinee:

19. _____
    _____
20. _____
21. _____
22. _____
23. _____
24. _____
25. _____
26. _____
27. _____

SP CHECKLIST FOR MR. SULLIVAN

History of Present Illness. The Examinee:

____ 1. asked how long I have been experiencing the insomnia ("Almost 6 months now.")

____ 2. asked how many hours I sleep at night ("Maybe 2 hours every night.")

____ 3. asked if I have difficulty falling asleep ("No; I fall asleep immediately.")

____ 4. asked if I have difficulty staying asleep ("Yes; nightmares wake me up.")

____ 5. asked me to talk about my nightmares ("Vietnam; my entire platoon was killed during a raid except for me; I saw it happen.")

____ 6. asked me if I had feelings of guilt about surviving in Vietnam ("Yes.")

____ 7. asked me if I had flashbacks about the trauma I saw in Vietnam ("I can't get the thoughts out of my head. I relive the war, whether I want to or not, every day.")

____ 8. asked me about feelings of depression, i.e., hopelessness, sadness, loss of energy, inability to concentrate ("Yes; I have all of those.")

____ 9. asked me if I was emotionally distant from people ("My wife left me because of that.")

____ 10. asked me if I have withdrawn from all activities ("Yes; I stay home all day; I even lost my job.")

____ 11. asked about any periods of violence ("I hit my wife; that is why she left me. My temper is unpredictable. I was arrested for fighting a couple of times.")

____ 12. asked me if I felt anxious much of the time ("Yes; sometimes a car backfiring will cause me to jump up in fear. It sounds like a gunshot.")

____ 13. asked me if I use tobacco ("I smoke 3 packs of cigarettes a day.")

____ 14. asked me if I drink alcohol ("Maybe 2 beers a day.")

____ 15. asked me if I use illicit drugs ("No.")

____ 16. asked if I take any medications ("No.")

____ 17. asked if I have ever been ill before ("No illnesses.")

____ 18. asked about a family history of psychiatric problems ("No.")

Communication Skills. The Examinee:

____ 19. explained the initial diagnostic possibilities with me (i.e., posttraumatic stress disorder, depression, mood disorder).

____ 20. explained that it is possible for this to occur many years after a traumatic event.

____ 21. explained that my violence was part of the disorder.

____ 22. explained that I would need medication.

____ 23. explained that I would need therapy (group and behavioral therapy).

____ 24. offered me ongoing support.

____ 25. addressed my nonverbal reactions (tearfulness).

____ 26. reassured me that I would improve.

____ 27. conveyed a sense of confidence.

If you performed 19 of these 27 tasks, you passed this test station.

You have 10 minutes to complete your patient note.

HISTORY—Include significant positives and negatives from the history of present illness, past medical history, review of systems, and social and family history.

_____
_____
_____
_____
_____
_____
_____
_____
_____
_____

PHYSICAL EXAMINATION—Indicate only the pertinent positive and negative findings related to the patient's chief complaint.

_____
_____
_____
_____
_____
_____
_____
_____
_____
_____

DIFFERENTIAL DIAGNOSIS—In order of likelihood, write no more than five differential diagnoses for this patient's current problems.

1. _____
2. _____
3. _____
4. _____
5. _____

DIAGNOSTIC WORKUP—Immediate plans for no more than five diagnostic studies.

1. _____
2. _____
3. _____
4. _____
5. _____

A SATISFACTORY PATIENT NOTE

HISTORY—Include significant positives and negatives from the history of present illness, past medical history, review of systems, and social and family history.

Fifty-year-old Mr. Albert Sullivan presents with a 6-month history of insomnia. He has no difficulty falling asleep but awakens after 2 hours with nightmares centered around his wartime experiences in Vietnam. His entire platoon was killed during a raid and he was the only survivor. Mr. Sullivan feels guilty about surviving the trauma. He is plagued by recurring thoughts about the event in the form of flashbacks and nightmares. He feels anxious most of the time and is easily frightened by sounds that remind him of his wartime experience. He has feelings of hopelessness and sadness. He is unable to concentrate and lacks energy. He feels emotionally distant and withdrawn. He is prone to violent outbursts and aggressive behavior and has been arrested for fighting. His divorce was the result of spousal abuse. He has lost his job recently and is at home all day. He smokes three packs of cigarettes per day and drinks 2 beers a day. He does not take medications or abuse illicit drugs. He has no past medical illnesses. Psychiatric problems do not run in his family.

PHYSICAL EXAMINATION—Indicate only the pertinent positive and negative findings related to the patient's chief complaint.

T = 98.7°F. BP = 115/75 mmHg. HR = 80 beats/min. RR = 12 breaths/min.
The patient is a well-developed well-nourished male in NAD. He appears to be on edge and extremely anxious. He is guarded when answering questions. He often raises his voice and angers easily.

DIFFERENTIAL DIAGNOSIS
In order of likelihood, write no more than five differential diagnoses for this patient's current problems.

1. posttraumatic stress disorder
2. major depression
3. mood disorder
4. anxiety disorder
5. substance abuse

DIAGNOSTIC WORKUP
Immediate plans for no more than five diagnostic studies.

1. behavioral therapy
2. group therapy
3. urine toxicology
4.
5.

LEARNING OBJECTIVE FOR MR. SULLIVAN
EVALUATE THE PATIENT WHO PRESENTS WITH INSOMNIA

Mr. Sullivan presents with the chief complaint of insomnia. On further questioning, it becomes clear that the patient is unable to remain asleep because of nightmares. As a soldier in Vietnam, Mr. Sullivan witnessed the violent death of his entire platoon; 25 years later, he is suffering from PTSD.

PTSD may occur shortly or decades after a person has experienced or witnessed a violent, traumatizing event. The symptoms of this disorder include anxiety and depression. The patient is withdrawn and distant from loved ones. The patient feels guilty about having survived the trauma. He is plagued by recurring thoughts about the event in the form of flashbacks and nightmares.

Mr. Sullivan is prone to aggressive behavior and violent outbursts. He has been arrested for fighting and admits to spousal abuse. He is easily frightened by sounds that remind him of his wartime experience. These are symptoms of PTSD.

The trauma causing PTSD must be of great magnitude (assault, motor vehicle accident, torture, fire, war, or natural disaster experience).

The treatment of PTSD includes behavioral therapy, group therapy, and the use of medications [anxiolytics, beta blockers, α-adrenergic agonists, selective serotonin reuptake inhibitors (SSRIs)]. Even with intensive therapy, 50 percent of patients with PTSD have a chronic, persistent illness.

History-Taking Pearl: PTSD may develop within 1 week or as long as 30 years after the traumatic event (often the case in victims of child abuse).

Difficulty sleeping is a common chief complaint, and the examinee should differentiate between insomnia ("I can't sleep"), hypersomnia ("I sleep too much, especially during the day"), and parasomnia ("My wife says I do unusual things when I sleep"). A person with insomnia should be asked whether he or she has difficulty falling asleep or staying asleep.

Patient Note Pearl: The **differential diagnosis** of PTSD includes major depression, mood disorder, malingering, and anxiety disorder. Substance abuse must be excluded as an etiology for the patient's behavior. The **diagnostic workup** might include behavioral and group therapy along with response to medication use.

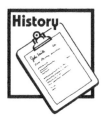

Case 46

A 52-year-old woman, Ms. Mary Meany, presents to the emergency room complaining of severe abdominal pain. You enter the examination room and observe an obese woman lying on a stretcher squirming in pain. She appears to be uncomfortable and in some distress. The rectal examination performed by your physician assistant revealed no masses; stool was brown in color and negative for occult blood.

Vital Signs:

Temperature	100.7°F
Blood pressure	120/80 mmHg
Heart rate	110 beats per minute
Respiratory rate	14 breaths per minute

Examinee's Tasks
(Do not repeat rectal examination)

1. Obtain a focused and relevant history.
2. Obtain a focused and relevant physical examination.
3. Discuss your initial diagnostic impressions with the patient.
4. Discuss follow-up tests with the patient.
5. After seeing the patient, complete paperwork relevant to the case.

MY CHECKLIST

History of Present Illness. The Examinee:

1. _____
2. _____
3. _____
4. _____
5. _____
6. _____
7. _____
8. _____
9. _____
10. _____
11. _____
12. _____
13. _____
14. _____
15. _____
16. _____

Physical Examination. The Examinee:

17. _____
18. _____
19. _____
20. _____

Communication Skills. The Examinee:

21. _____
22. _____
23. _____
24. _____
25. _____

SP CHECKLIST FOR MS. MEANY

History of Present Illness. The Examinee:

___ 1. asked about the location of the pain ("It's on the right side under my ribs.")
___ 2. asked about the onset of the pain ("It started 4 hours ago.")
___ 3. asked about the progression of the pain ("It seems to be getting worse.")
___ 4. asked about the quality of the pain ("It feels like a big crampy pain.")
___ 5. asked about the intensity of the pain ("On a scale of 1 to 10, this is a 10.")
___ 6. asked about the radiation of the pain ("It goes to my right shoulder.")
___ 7. asked about any aggravating factors ("Deep breath, fatty foods, and water make it worse.")
___ 8. asked about any alleviating factors ("None that I can think of.")
___ 9. asked about any previous episodes ("Last year this happened but it went away after 2 hours.")
___10. asked about any nausea and vomiting ("Yes. I vomited once and I still feel nauseated.")
___11. asked about any fever ("I haven't had time to check.")
___12. asked about any change in bowel movements ("No diarrhea or constipation.")
___13. asked about any blood in my stools or vomit ("None.")
___14. asked about my past medical history ("None.")
___15. asked about any alcohol use ("None.")
___16. asked about my diet ("Fatty and greasy foods.")

Physical Examination. The Examinee:

___17. listened with a stethoscope over my abdomen (normal bowel sounds auscultated).
___18. tapped over my liver to measure size (liver 12 cm MCL).
___19. pressed deeply over my abdomen (SP will complain of severe right-sided pain under ribs).
___20. tried to elicit a Murphy's sign (positive pain with deep breath when right side is pressed).

Communication Skills. The Examinee:

___21. acknowledged my discomfort during the physical examination.
___22. explained the initial diagnostic possibilities with me (i.e., cholecystitis, ulcer disease, pancreatitis).
___23. discussed the plan with me (blood work, ultrasonography, and possible surgery).
___24. discussed the prognosis (excellent).
___25. addressed my concerns about the surgery.

If you performed 18 of these 25 tasks, you passed this test station.

You have 10 minutes to complete your patient note.

HISTORY—Include significant positives and negatives from the history of present illness, past medical history, review of systems, and social and family history.

_____
_____
_____
_____
_____
_____
_____
_____
_____
_____

PHYSICAL EXAMINATION—Indicate only the pertinent positive and negative findings related to the patient's chief complaint.

_____
_____
_____
_____
_____
_____
_____
_____
_____
_____

DIFFERENTIAL DIAGNOSIS—In order of likelihood, write no more than five differential diagnoses for this patient's current problems.

1. _____
2. _____
3. _____
4. _____
5. _____

DIAGNOSTIC WORKUP—Immediate plans for no more than five diagnostic studies.

1. _____
2. _____
3. _____
4. _____
5. _____

A SATISFACTORY PATIENT NOTE

HISTORY—Include significant positives and negatives from the history of present illness, past medical history, review of systems, and social and family history.

Ms. Mary Meany, an obese, 52-year-old woman, presents with a 4-hour history of severe crampy right-upper-quadrant pain that radiates to her right shoulder and is accompanied by nausea and vomiting. She describes the pain as a 10 on a scale of 1 to 10. Deep breathing, fatty foods, and water worsen the pain; nothing alleviates the pain. She denies having fever, hematemesis, or a change in bowel movements. She states that similar symptoms occurred last year but they resolved without medical attention. She has never been ill and denies tobacco and alcohol use. Her diet consists mainly of greasy and fatty foods.

PHYSICAL EXAMINATION—Indicate only the pertinent positive and negative findings related to the patient's chief complaint.

T = 100.7°F. BP = 120/80 mmHg. HR = 110 beats/min. RR = 14 breaths/min.
The patient is an obese woman lying on a stretcher and squirming in pain. She appears to be uncomfortable and in some distress.
Skin: No jaundice. Negative Turner's and Cullen's signs.
Heart: Normal S_1 and S_2. No murmurs, rubs, or gallops.
Lungs: Clear to auscultation.
Abdomen: Normal BS. Liver size MCL 12 cm by percussion. Severe RUQ tenderness with palpation. +Murphy's sign. No ascites.
Rectal Examination: No masses or tenderness. FOBT negative.

DIFFERENTIAL DIAGNOSIS
In order of likelihood, write no more than five differential diagnoses for this patient's current problems.

1. cholecystitis
2. pancreatitis
3. appendicitis
4. peptic ulcer disease
5. hepatitis

DIAGNOSTIC WORKUP
Immediate plans for no more than five diagnostic studies.

1. CBC with differential
2. abdominal ultrasound
3. AST and ALT
4. alkaline phosphatase and bilirubin
5. amylase and lipase

LEARNING OBJECTIVE FOR MS. MEANY
APPROACH TO THE PATIENT WITH RIGHT-UPPER-QUADRANT PAIN

Ms. Meany is an obese woman who presents with severe right-upper-quadrant pain that radiates to her right shoulder and is accompanied by nausea and vomiting. She states that similar symptoms occurred last year but they resolved without medical attention. She denies having hematemesis or a change in bowel movements. She is not a diabetic. On presentation, she has a low-grade fever and is mildly tachycardic.

The patient denies alcohol use. Her diet consists of fatty and greasy food. The differential diagnosis after obtaining the history on this patient includes acute cholecystitis, pancreatitis, appendicitis, and ulcer disease.

On physical examination, the patient has severe right-upper-quadrant pain on palpation and a positive Murphy's sign. The gallbladder is not palpable. The most likely diagnosis after the physical examination is acute cholecystitis.

The workup for this patient includes a white blood cell count looking for the leukocytosis that often accompanies cholecystitis. Liver function test results and pancreatic enzymes may also be elevated. Ultrasonography will visualize the gallbladder stones and identify changes seen with acute cholecystitis, such as thickening of the gallbladder wall. Surgery is indicated in this patient, and her prognosis is excellent.

Patient Note Pearl: The **differential diagnosis** for this patient would be cholecystitis, pancreatitis, ulcer disease, hepatitis, and appendicitis. The **diagnostic workup** would include a CBC, aspartate aminotransferase (AST), alanine aminotransferase (ALT), alkaline phosphatase, bilirubin levels, amylase, lipase, and abdominal ultrasound.

Case 47

Tommy Trucker is a 35-year-old tractor-trailer driver who presents to the emergency room complaining of severe left-sided back pain. The patient will not lie down on the examination table and is demanding pain medication. You enter the room and find the patient pacing up and down. He is tilted to one side. He sees you and immediately asks for pain medications. He is threatening to go to another hospital if pain medications continue to be withheld. He is 6 feet tall and weighs approximately 250 pounds. He has snake tattoos on his arms and left cheek. Rectal examination and examination of the genitalia were performed by the physician assistant and were normal.

Vital Signs:

Temperature   98.9°F
Blood pressure   135/80 mmHg
Heart rate   100 beats per minute
Respiratory rate   14 breaths per minute

Examinee's Tasks
(Do not repeat genitalia or rectal examinations)

1. Obtain a focused and relevant history.
2. Obtain a focused and relevant physical examination.
3. Discuss your initial diagnostic impressions with the patient.
4. Discuss follow-up tests with the patient.
5. After seeing the patient, complete paperwork relevant to the case.

MY CHECKLIST

History of Present Illness. The Examinee:

1. _____
2. _____
3. _____
4. _____
5. _____
6. _____
7. _____
8. _____
9. _____
10. _____
11. _____
12. _____
13. _____
14. _____

Physical Examination. The Examinee:

15. _____
16. _____
17. _____
    _____
18. _____
    _____

Communication Skills. The Examinee:

19. _____
20. _____
21. _____
22. _____
23. _____
24. _____

SP CHECKLIST FOR MR. TRUCKER

History of Present Illness. The Examinee:

___ 1. asked about the location of the pain ("The entire left part of my back and side; it comes and goes.")

___ 2. asked about the onset of the pain ("It started about 3 hours ago.")

___ 3. asked about the quality of the pain ("It is like someone is punching me in the side.")

___ 4. asked about the progression of the pain ("It is getting worse; I need pain medications.")

___ 5. asked about any radiation of the pain ("It seems to be going into my left groin area.")

___ 6. asked about any association with nausea or vomiting ("No.")

___ 7. asked about any change in my bowel movements ("No.")

___ 8. asked about any blood in my stool ("None.")

___ 9. asked about any urinary complaints, e.g., dysuria, frequency ("None.")

___10. asked about any blood in my urine ("It did look a little bloody earlier this morning.")

___11. asked about any trauma to the area ("No.")

___12. asked if this pain has ever occurred before ("No.")

___13. asked about any alcohol use ("Maybe a couple of beers a day.")

___14. asked about any drug use ("Just some marijuana now and then.")

Physical Examination. The Examinee:

___15. listened to my abdomen with a stethoscope (normal bowel sounds).

___16. pressed deeply over my abdomen (no pain is elicited).

___17. tapped on the left side of my back for any costovertebral angle tenderness (SP will jump off the examination table in pain).

___18. performed a musculoskeletal examination of my back, i.e., range of motion, straight leg raising (normal examination of back; SP can bend in all directions easily).

Communication Skills. The Examinee:

___19. acknowledged my distress and discomfort.

___20. did not become frustrated or angry with me.

___21. discussed the diagnostic possibilities with me (i.e., kidney stone, pyelonephritis).

___22. explained the importance of a urine sample to check for blood in the urine.

___23. explained the workup to me (blood work, urinalysis, abdominal radiograph, urology consultation).

___24. told me I will receive pain medications.

If you performed 17 of these 24 tasks, you passed this test station.

You have 10 minutes to complete your patient note.

HISTORY—Include significant positives and negatives from the history of present illness, past medical history, review of systems, and social and family history.

_____
_____
_____
_____
_____
_____
_____
_____
_____
_____

PHYSICAL EXAMINATION—Indicate only the pertinent positive and negative findings related to the patient's chief complaint.

_____
_____
_____
_____
_____
_____
_____
_____
_____
_____

DIFFERENTIAL DIAGNOSIS—In order of likelihood, write no more than five differential diagnoses for this patient's current problems.

1. _____
2. _____
3. _____
4. _____
5. _____

DIAGNOSTIC WORKUP—Immediate plans for no more than five diagnostic studies.

1. _____
2. _____
3. _____
4. _____
5. _____

A SATISFACTORY PATIENT NOTE

HISTORY—Include significant positives and negatives from the history of present illness, past medical history, review of systems, and social and family history.

Mr. Tommy Trucker is a 35-year-old truck driver who presents to the emergency room complaining of severe left-sided flank pain that radiates to his back and left groin. The pain started suddenly 3 hours ago, is colicky in nature, and has been worsening progressively. Mr. Trucker describes the pain as like someone punching him in the back; it is so severe that he is requesting pain medication. He denies nausea, vomiting, diarrhea, constipation or bloody stools. He has no urinary complaints and denies hematuria. He has no past history of similar pain and denies trauma to the back or groin. He drinks two beers per day and smokes marijuana occasionally.

PHYSICAL EXAMINATION—Indicate only the pertinent positive and negative findings related to the patient's chief complaint.

T = 98.9°F. BP = 135/80 mmHg. HR = 100 beats/min. RR = 14 breaths/min. Ht = 6 ft. Wt = 250 lb.
The patient is an anxious 35-year-old man who will not lie down on the examination table. He is pacing up and down and tilted to one side. He is threatening to go to another hospital if pain medications continue to be withheld.
Skin: Snake tattoos on both arms and left cheek.
Heart: Normal S_1 and S_2.
Lungs: Clear to auscultation.
Abdomen: Normal BS. Nontender. Positive left CVA tenderness.
Rectal Examination: No masses. Nontender. FOBT negative.
Genitalia: Normal examination.
Musculoskeletal: Back with full ROM. Normal straight leg raise maneuver.

DIFFERENTIAL DIAGNOSIS
In order of likelihood, write no more than five differential diagnoses for this patient's current problems.

1. kidney stone
2. pyelonephritis
3. testicular torsion
4. epididymitis
5. musculoskeletal pain

DIAGNOSTIC WORKUP
Immediate plans for no more than five diagnostic studies.

1. urinalysis
2. CBC
3. plain film of the abdomen
4. electrolytes
5. BUN and creatinine

LEARNING OBJECTIVE FOR MR. TRUCKER
APPROACH TO THE PATIENT WITH FLANK PAIN AND HEMATURIA

Mr. Trucker presents with severe left-sided flank pain that radiates to his back and groin area. He has some hematuria. He denies having a history of trauma to the area or any back injury. He is demanding pain medications, and the staff suspects that he is seeking drugs.

You are asked to evaluate the patient and realize that his symptomatology is consistent with kidney stones even though the patient denies having had previous painful episodes (kidney stones are recurrent). He denies having any gastrointestinal and other urinary complaints. The abdominal and inguinal examinations are normal. There is no evidence of an acute abdomen, testicular torsion, or epididymitis. Examination of the back reveals no musculoskeletal physical findings. There is, however, left costovertebral angle tenderness, which is consistent with pyelonephritis or a kidney stone. Since the patient is afebrile, kidney stone is the more likely possibility. A urinalysis of this patient might reveal microscopic hematuria without nitrites or leukocytes. The abdominal radiograph may show the kidney stones in the left ureter. The treatment for kidney stones is vigorous hydration and analgesics. Renal function tests should be followed closely, and a workup for the etiology of his stones will be initiated [stones may contain calcium oxalate (35 percent), calcium apatite (35 percent), magnesium ammonium phosphate or struvite (20 percent), uric acid (5 percent), or cystine (2–3 percent)]. Most kidney stones will pass spontaneously.

You should be open-minded and nonjudgmental in evaluating this patient. You should elicit the appropriate history and perform the necessary physical examination on this demanding patient in order to arrive at the correct diagnosis.

History-Taking Pearl: Hematuria is a common chief complaint. If your doctor does not know the mnemonic for hematuria, **SWITCH GPs** (switch general practitioners):

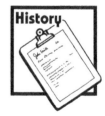

S = stones, sickle cell disease, sickle cell trait, scleroderma, SLE, schistosomiasis, and sulfonamides

W = Wegener's granulomatosis

I = infections, instrumentation, iatrogenic (analgesics, anticoagulants, and cyclophosphamide), interstitial nephritis

T = trauma, tuberculosis, tubulointerstitial disease, tumor, and thrombotic thrombocytopenic purpura

C = cryoglobulinemia

H = hemolytic-uremic syndrome, hypercalciuria, hemophilia, and Henoch-Schönlein purpura

G = Goodpasture's disease, glomerulonephritis

P = papillary necrosis, polycystic kidney disease, and polyarteritis nodosa

S = sponge disease (medullary sponge disease)

Patient Note Pearl: The **differential diagnosis** for this patient includes kidney stones, pyelonephritis, testicular torsion, epididymitis, and musculoskeletal pain. The **diagnostic workup** would include a CBC, urinalysis, and a plain film of the abdomen. All first-time kidney stone patients should have blood work sent for electrolytes, BUN, creatinine, calcium, phosphate, and uric acid levels. Twenty-four-hour urine collections for calcium, uric acid, phosphate, oxalate, and citrate are requested in patients with recurrent stones or with a positive family history.

NOTES

Case 48

You are asked to evaluate Mr. Johnny Guitar, a 50-year-old musician in the emergency room complaining of abdominal pain. The patient was originally triaged to the nonurgent area of the emergency room for treatment of food poisoning, but the intern working in that area feels something more is going on. You are the consulting physician. The intern informs you that the rectal examination was normal but he could not do a FOBT due to lack of stool in the vault. Examination of the genitalia revealed no hernias or masses.

Vital Signs:

Temperature	100.5°F
Blood pressure	110/70 mmHg
Heart rate	112 beats per minute
Respiratory rate	22 breaths per minute

Examinee's Tasks
(Do not repeat the rectal and genitalia examinations)

1. Obtain a focused and relevant history.
2. Obtain a focused and relevant physical examination.
3. Discuss your initial diagnostic impressions with the patient.
4. Discuss follow-up tests with the patient.
5. After seeing the patient, complete paperwork relevant to the case.

MY CHECKLIST

History of Present Illness. The Examinee:

1. _____
2. _____
   _____
3. _____
4. _____
5. _____
6. _____
7. _____
8. _____
9. _____
10. _____
11. _____
12. _____

Physical Examination. The Examinee:

13. _____
14. _____
15. _____
    _____
16. _____
17. _____

Communication Skills. The Examinee:

18. _____
19. _____
20. _____
21. _____
22. _____
23. _____
24. _____

SP CHECKLIST FOR MR. GUITAR

History of Present Illness. The Examinee:

___ 1.   asked about the location of the pain ("No special area; It's all over my abdomen.")

___ 2.   asked about the quality of the pain ("It is crampy and colicky; in music it would be called crescendo-decrescendo.")

___ 3.   asked about the frequency of the pain ("It comes every 10 minutes or so.")

___ 4.   asked about the duration of the pain ("It lasts maybe 1 minute, then eases off, like a contraction in labor.")

___ 5.   asked about the onset of the pain ("Started yesterday.")

___ 6.   asked about any nausea or vomiting ("Vomited 8 times since last night.")

___ 7.   asked about any blood in the vomitus ("No.")

___ 8.   asked about any change in bowel movements ("Have not had a bowel movement for 2 days.")

___ 9.   asked about passing any flatus ("None.")

___10.   asked about any fever ("None.")

___11.   asked about any weight loss ("None.")

___12.   asked about my past surgical history ("I had an appendectomy at the age of 22.")

Physical Examination. The Examinee:

___13.   listened to my abdomen with a stethoscope (increased bowel sounds).

___14.   tapped or percussed over my abdomen (positive tympany).

___15.   palpated gently over my abdomen (SP will guard the abdomen and complain of diffuse pain with gentle palpation).

___16.   palpated deeply over my abdomen (SP will complain of severe pain with deep palpation).

___17.   tried to elicit rebound tenderness (no rebound tenderness).

Communication Skills. The Examinee:

___18.   discussed the initial diagnostic possibilities with me (i.e., intestinal obstruction, paralytic ileus).

___19.   explained that the cause of an obstruction would be the adhesions from my previous surgery.

___20.   explained the plan (blood work, abdominal radiography, intravenous fluids, nasogastric tube).

___21.   explained the prognosis (excellent).

___22.   showed consideration for my discomfort.

___23.   addressed my concerns about the nasogastric tube.

___24.   was reassuring.

If you performed 17 of these 24 tasks, you passed this test station.

You have 10 minutes to complete your patient note.

HISTORY—Include significant positives and negatives from the history of present illness, past medical history, review of systems, and social and family history.

_____

_____

_____

_____

_____

_____

_____

_____

_____

_____

PHYSICAL EXAMINATION—Indicate only the pertinent positive and negative findings related to the patient's chief complaint.

_____

_____

_____

_____

_____

_____

_____

_____

_____

_____

DIFFERENTIAL DIAGNOSIS—In order of likelihood, write no more than five differential diagnoses for this patient's current problems.

1. _____

2. _____

3. _____

4. _____

5. _____

DIAGNOSTIC WORKUP—Immediate plans for no more than five diagnostic studies.

1. _____

2. _____

3. _____

4. _____

5. _____

A SATISFACTORY PATIENT NOTE

HISTORY—Include significant positives and negatives from the history of present illness, past medical history, review of systems, and social and family history.

> Mr. Johnny Guitar, 50 years old, presents with a 1-day history of diffuse abdominal pain accompanied by profuse vomiting. The pain is colicky in nature, coming in 10-minute intervals and lasting 1 minute. He is not passing any stool or flatus. He denies fever and recent weight loss. He has a surgical history of appendectomy at the age of 22.

PHYSICAL EXAMINATION—Indicate only the pertinent positive and negative findings related to the patient's chief complaint.

> T = 100.5°F. BP = 110/70 mmHg. HR = 112 beats/min. RR = 22 breaths/min.
> The patient is a well-developed well-nourished male who is in moderate distress when he develops bouts of abdominal pain. When pain-free he is comfortable and in NAD.
> **Heart:** Normal S_1 and S_2.
> **Lungs:** Clear to auscultation.
> **Abdomen:** Positive appendectomy scar. Increased BS. + Guarding. No rigidity. + Tympany. Diffuse tenderness with palpation. No rebound tenderness.
> **Rectal Examination:** No masses. Nontender. No stool in vault.
> **Genitalia:** Normal examination. No hernias present.

DIFFERENTIAL DIAGNOSIS	DIAGNOSTIC WORKUP
In order of likelihood, write no more than five differential diagnoses for this patient's current problems.	Immediate plans for no more than five diagnostic studies.
1. intestinal obstruction	1. CBC with differential
2. ileus	2. electrolytes
3. mesenteric ischemia	3. abdominal radiograph
4. pancreatitis	4. BUN and creatinine
5. gastroenteritis	5. rectal examination with FOBT

LEARNING OBJECTIVE FOR MR. GUITAR

EVALUATE THE PATIENT WHO PRESENTS WITH COLICKY ABDOMINAL PAIN

Mr. Guitar presents with complaints of diffuse colicky abdominal pain and profuse vomiting. He is not passing any stool or flatus. Mr. Guitar had an appendectomy over 25 years ago; with this surgical history, he is at risk for small bowel obstruction secondary to adhesions. Other etiologies for small bowel obstruction include an incarcerated hernia, a stricture due to IBD, and a malignancy (large bowel obstruction may be due to malignancy, fecal impaction, volvulus, and diverticulitis). An abdominal radiograph will demonstrate the lack of air in the rectum and the ladder-like pattern of a dilated small bowel with air-fluid levels. A nasogastric tube should be inserted immediately to reduce any distention proximal to the obstruction and relieve the vomiting. Intravenous fluid support is required, and electrolytes should be monitored for evidence of dehydration. Strangulation with bowel necrosis is a complication of obstruction and may lead to perforation and sepsis. Mr. Guitar requires surgery to relieve the obstruction.

Patient Note Pearl: The **differential diagnosis** for this patient includes intestinal obstruction, paralytic ileus (no bowel sounds on physical examination), mesenteric ischemia, ileus, pancreatitis, and gastroenteritis. The **diagnostic workup** would include a rectal examination with FOBT, CBC, analysis of electrolytes, and an abdominal radiograph.

Case 49

You are asked by the geriatrician to consult on a 77-year-old man named Thomas Toomer, who was admitted to the geriatrics service a few hours ago for acute onset of abdominal pain. The geriatrician reports that the rectal examination was FOBT-positive; no masses were palpable in the cul-de-sac.

Vital Signs:

Temperature	101.6°F
Blood pressure	100/70 mmHg
Heart rate	120 beats per minute
Respirations	22 breaths per minute

Examinee's Tasks
(Do not repeat the rectal examination)

1. Obtain a focused and relevant history.
2. Obtain a focused and relevant physical examination.
3. Discuss your initial diagnostic impressions with the patient.
4. Discuss follow-up tests with the patient.
5. After seeing the patient, complete paperwork relevant to the case.

MY CHECKLIST

History of Present Illness. The Examinee:

1. _____
2. _____
3. _____
4. _____
5. _____
6. _____
7. _____
8. _____
9. _____
10. _____
11. _____
12. _____
13. _____
14. _____
15. _____
16. _____
17. _____

Physical Examination. The Examinee:

18. _____
19. _____
20. _____
21. _____

Communication Skills. The Examinee:

22. _____
23. _____
    _____
24. _____
25. _____
26. _____
27. _____

SP CHECKLIST FOR MR. TOOMER

History of Present Illness. The Examinee:

___ 1. asked about the location of the pain ("It's in the left lower side of my abdomen.")

___ 2. asked about the onset of the pain ("It's been going on for 36 to 48 hours.")

___ 3. asked about the quality of the pain ("Crampy. Do you think I'll need surgery, Doc?")

___ 4. asked about the frequency of the pain ("It's happening every 15 minutes. Like I'm having a baby.")

___ 5. asked about the progression of the pain ("It seems to be getting stronger.")

___ 6. asked about the radiation of the pain ("It stays on the left lower side.")

___ 7. asked about any aggravating factors ("Nothing I can think of.")

___ 8. asked about any alleviating factors ("Nothing makes it better. Will I need surgery to make it better?")

___ 9. asked about any fever ("At home, it was 102°F. I also had chills; does that mean I need an operation?")

___10. asked about any nausea and vomiting ("None.")

___11. asked about a change in bowel movements ("I am having a little diarrhea.")

___12. asked about any blood in my stools ("None.")

___13. asked about any urinary complaints, i.e., frequency, dysuria ("No.")

___14. asked about my diet ("I eat junk food; no fruits, cereals, or vegetables.")

___15. asked about weight loss ("None.")

___16. asked about alcohol abuse ("I drink one beer a week.")

___17. asked about tobacco use ("No cigarettes.")

Physical Examination. The Examinee:

___18. listened to my abdomen with a stethoscope (normal bowel sounds auscultated).

___19. pressed gently on my abdomen (tenderness when pressing left lower side of my abdomen).

___20. pressed deeply on my abdomen (severe tenderness when pressing left lower side).

___21. attempted to elicit rebound tenderness (positive rebound tenderness when letting go of left lower side).

Communication Skills. The Examinee:

___22. explained the initial impression to me (diverticulitis, colitis, abscess in my colon).

___23. explained the workup (rectal examination, intravenous fluids, blood work, radiographs, nasogastric tube, antibiotics).

___24. explained that conservative management would be tried before any surgery.

___25. stated that surgery may still be necessary.

___26. addressed my concerns about any surgery.

___27. offered understanding of my emotions.

If you performed 19 of these 27 tasks, you passed this test station.

You have 10 minutes to complete your patient note.

HISTORY—Include significant positives and negatives from the history of present illness, past medical history, review of systems, and social and family history.

_____
_____
_____
_____
_____
_____
_____
_____
_____
_____

PHYSICAL EXAMINATION—Indicate only the pertinent positive and negative findings related to the patient's chief complaint.

_____
_____
_____
_____
_____
_____
_____
_____
_____
_____

DIFFERENTIAL DIAGNOSIS—In order of likelihood, write no more than five differential diagnoses for this patient's current problems.

1. _____
2. _____
3. _____
4. _____
5. _____

DIAGNOSTIC WORKUP—Immediate plans for no more than five diagnostic studies.

1. _____
2. _____
3. _____
4. _____
5. _____

A SATISFACTORY PATIENT NOTE

HISTORY—Include significant positives and negatives from the history of present illness, past medical history, review of systems, and social and family history.

Mr. Thomas Toomer is a 77-year-old man with a 2-day history of crampy LLQ pain that is intermittent in nature and progressively worsening. The pain does not radiate and is associated with mild diarrhea. At home he had a fever to 102°F and shaking chills. Nothing he does alleviates the pain and nothing makes the pain worse. He denies constipation, nausea, vomiting, bloody stools, and urinary complaints. He has no weight loss. His diet consists of mostly junk food; he does not eat fruits, vegetables, or cereals. He has never been ill before and takes no medications. He does not smoke cigarettes or drink alcohol.

PHYSICAL EXAMINATION—Indicate only the pertinent positive and negative findings related to the patient's chief complaint.

T = 101.6°F. BP = 100/70 mmHg. HR = 120 beats/min. RR = 22 breaths/min.
The patient is fearful and ill-looking. He is in moderate distress.
Skin: Warm to touch. Diaphoretic
Heart: S_1 and S_2 normal. Tachycardia.
Lungs: Clear to auscultation.
Abdomen: +BS. Severe tenderness LLQ. +Rebound tenderness.
Rectal Examination: No masses palpable in cul-de-sac. FOBT +.

DIFFERENTIAL DIAGNOSIS
In order of likelihood, write no more than five differential diagnoses for this patient's current problems.

1. diverticulitis
2. appendicitis
3. ischemic colitis
4. colon cancer
5.

DIAGNOSTIC WORKUP
Immediate plans for no more than five diagnostic studies.

1. CBC with differential
2. abdominal film
3. CT scan of the abdomen
4. electrolytes
5. BUN and creatinine

LEARNING OBJECTIVE FOR MR. TOOMER
APPROACH TO AN ELDERLY PATIENT
WITH LOWER ABDOMINAL PAIN AND FEVER

Mr. Thomas Toomer is an elderly gentleman who presents with crampy left-lower-quadrant pain associated with mild diarrhea. He is febrile and tachycardic. He denies having nausea, vomiting, or urinary complaints. He dislikes physicians and has a great fear of surgery. He has been at home for 2 days trying on his own to get well in an effort to avoid a hospital admission.

On physical examination, Mr. Toomer has severe tenderness with rebound on palpation of the left lower quadrant. Blood work will reveal a leukocytosis and radiographic studies may reveal free air, ileus, or an abdominal mass. A CT study of the abdomen may reveal a collection in the colon consistent with an abscess. Diverticulitis is the most plausible diagnosis in this patient.

Conservative treatment with intravenous hydration, nasogastric suctioning, and antibiotics may be attempted on this patient, but if improvement does not occur, surgical drainage or resection of the infected area is required. The patient should increase the fiber in his diet after discharge in an effort to prevent future episodes of diverticulitis. Even with dietary change, recurrent bouts of diverticulitis are common.

Patient Note Pearl: The **differential diagnosis** for this patient includes diverticulitis, appendicitis, ischemic colitis, and colon cancer (perforated). Gynecologic disorders (i.e., ruptured ovarian cyst) must be considered in female patients. The **diagnostic workup** includes CBC, abdominal film and, if needed, a CT scan of the abdomen.

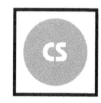

Case 50

A 32-year-old man named Markie Mackey was assaulted outside his home. He was hit several times in the stomach with a baseball bat. Although he stated that he was feeling fine, his wife is concerned and brings him to the emergency room. Rectal examination was performed by the nurse practitioner; there were no masses and stool was FOBT-negative.

Vital Signs:

Temperature	98.7°F
Blood pressure	100/70 mmHg
Heart rate	110 beats per minute
Respiratory rate	22 breaths per minute

Examinee's Tasks

1. Obtain a focused and relevant history.
2. Obtain a focused and relevant physical examination.
3. Discuss your initial diagnostic impressions with the patient.
4. Discuss follow-up tests with the patient.
5. After seeing the patient, complete paperwork relevant to the case.

MY CHECKLIST

History of Present Illness. The Examinee:

1. _____
2. _____
3. _____
4. _____
5. _____
6. _____
7. _____
8. _____

Physical Examination. The Examinee:

9. _____
_____
10. _____
11. _____
12. _____
13. _____
14. _____
15. _____
16. _____

Communication Skills. The Examinee:

17. _____
18. _____
19. _____
20. _____
21. _____
22. _____
23. _____
24. _____

SP CHECKLIST FOR MR. MACKEY

History of Present Illness. The Examinee:

___ 1. asked me if I was having any pain ("My stomach is a little sore.")

___ 2. asked me if the pain radiated ("It seems to be going up to my left shoulder for some reason.")

___ 3. asked me if I felt nauseated ("A little nauseated.")

___ 4. asked about loss of consciousness ("No, I was awake through the whole thing.")

___ 5. asked about other symptoms, i.e., chest pain, shortness of breath, dizziness ("No.")

___ 6. asked me about any past medical history ("Never ill before.")

___ 7. asked me about any medication use ("None.")

___ 8. asked me about any allergies ("None.")

Physical Examination. The Examinee:

___ 9. checked for orthostatic changes (systolic blood pressure decreases by 20 mmHg and heart rate increases by 20 beats per minute with standing or with legs dangling off the side of the bed).

___10. listened to my lungs in at least four places (normal lung examination; no evidence of pneumothorax).

___11. palpated my ribs (tenderness over ninth and tenth ribs on the left side).

___12. listened over my abdomen with a stethoscope (normal bowel signs audible).

___13. pressed gently throughout my abdomen (mild tenderness on palpation over the left upper side).

___14. pressed deeply throughout my abdomen (mild tenderness over the left upper side).

___15. attempted to elicit rebound tenderness (no rebound tenderness).

___16. examined my left shoulder (normal examination).

Communication Skills. The Examinee:

___17. explained to me that I may have some internal bleeding.

___18. explained that I may have ruptured my spleen or liver.

___19. explained the workup to me (blood work, radiographs, vigorous intravenous hydration, transfusions).

___20. told me I would need a needle in my abdomen to check for blood.

___21. explained that I may need surgery.

___22. explained that I would probably keep most of my spleen or liver.

___23. addressed my concerns.

___24. demonstrated empathy.

If you performed 17 of these 24 tasks, you passed this test station.

You have 10 minutes to complete your patient note.

HISTORY—Include significant positives and negatives from the history of present illness, past medical history, review of systems, and social and family history.

_____

_____

_____

_____

_____

_____

_____

_____

_____

_____

PHYSICAL EXAMINATION—Indicate only the pertinent positive and negative findings related to the patient's chief complaint.

_____

_____

_____

_____

_____

_____

_____

_____

_____

_____

DIFFERENTIAL DIAGNOSIS—In order of likelihood, write no more than five differential diagnoses for this patient's current problems.

1. _____

2. _____

3. _____

4. _____

5. _____

DIAGNOSTIC WORKUP—Immediate plans for no more than five diagnostic studies.

1. _____

2. _____

3. _____

4. _____

5. _____

A SATISFACTORY PATIENT NOTE

HISTORY—Include significant positives and negatives from the history of present illness, past medical history, review of systems, and social and family history.

Mr. Markie Mackey is a 32-year-old man who was assaulted several times with a baseball bat in the abdomen. He has abdominal "soreness" and left shoulder-strap pain accompanied by nausea but is otherwise asymptomatic. He denies chest pain, shortness of breath, or dizziness. He did not lose consciousness. He has no past medical history and takes no medications. He has no allergies.

PHYSICAL EXAMINATION—Indicate only the pertinent positive and negative findings related to the patient's chief complaint.

T = 98.7°F.
BP = 100/70 mmHg lying. BP = 80/50 mmHg standing.
HR = 110 beats/min. RR = 22 breaths/min.
Pale and diaphoretic male. Appears uncomfortable.
HEENT: Trachea midline.
Heart: Tachycardia. S_1 and S_2 normal.
Lungs: Clear to auscultation. No evidence of pneumothorax. Tenderness over 9th and 10th ribs.
Abdomen: Normal BS. Nondistended. Mild tenderness under left rib cage. No rebound tenderness.
Musculoskeletal: Left shoulder full ROM. No tenderness.
Rectal Examination: No tenderness or masses. FOBT negative.

DIFFERENTIAL DIAGNOSIS	DIAGNOSTIC WORKUP
In order of likelihood, write no more than five differential diagnoses for this patient's current problems.	Immediate plans for no more than five diagnostic studies.
1. splenic rupture	1. CT scan of abdomen
2. fractured ribs	2. CBC
3. liver laceration	3. diagnostic peritoneal lavage
4.	4. urinalysis
5.	5.

LEARNING OBJECTIVE FOR MR. MACKEY
EVALUATE THE PATIENT WITH BLUNT TRAUMA INJURY

Mr. Mackey was assaulted several times in the abdomen with a blunt instrument. Although he feels minimal discomfort, his wife insists that he be examined by a doctor. The patient is tachycardic and hypotensive, with orthostatic changes. These are signs of hypovolemia due to blood loss.

On inspection of the abdomen, there is no distention. The ribs over the spleen are tender to palpation and are most likely fractured. There is mild abdominal tenderness on palpation but no rebound. In trauma patients, percussion over the spleen may reveal an area of dullness, which is a sign of splenic enlargement from bleeding. These subtle physical findings can be seen with splenic rupture.

Occasionally, a splenic rupture may present with a palpable mass in the left upper quadrant, accompanied by clear signs of peritonitis.

Abdominal radiographs in this patient may show the fractured ribs or an enlarged spleen. In the stabilized patient, a CT scan can better evaluate the extent of the splenic injury.

This patient's hematocrit may fall rapidly, requiring blood transfusions and vigorous hydration for stabilization. Diagnostic peritoneal lavage (DPL) will demonstrate blood in the abdomen (not organ-specific, however), and the patient will require a laparotomy. A good surgeon will make every effort to preserve as much spleen as possible (splenorrhaphy).

History-Taking Pearl: A simple mnemonic for all trauma patients is **AMPLE:**

A = **A**llergies
M = current **M**edications
P = **P**ast medical history
L = **L**ast meal
E = **E**vents before the accident

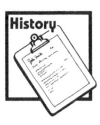

Physical Examination Pearl: Left shoulder-strap pain is often a classic finding in splenic rupture. This is called Kehr's sign.

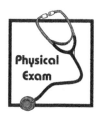

Patient Note Pearl: The **differential diagnosis** for this patient includes splenic rupture or liver laceration (can occur with blunt trauma; the liver establishes hemostasis quickly and may stop bleeding on its own without surgical intervention). The **diagnostic workup** includes CBC, DPL, urinalysis (for hematuria) and possibly a CT scan of the abdomen.

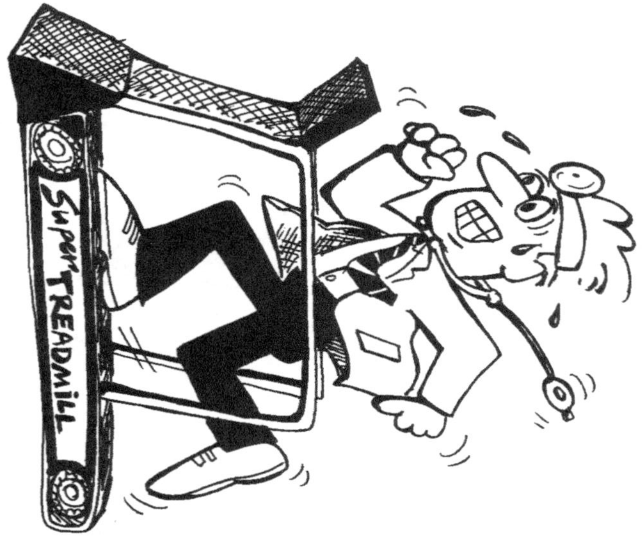

Section C: The Final Workout

Some Challenging Step 2 CS (Clinical Skills) Examination Cases

These three bonus cases are rated as difficult. If you find this final workout simple, you are adequately prepared for any Step 2 CS scenario. Congratulations!

Case 51: a 68-year-old woman with knee pain
Case 52: a 38-year-old man with anxiety
Case 53: a 44-year-old woman with weight loss and fatigue

Case 51

A 68-year-old woman named Olympia Ogelsby presents to your office complaining of left knee pain. She developed this while gambling in Atlantic City 2 days ago and went to the hotel doctor, who drained her knee. He gave her some pills and told her to see her doctor when she got home.

Vital Signs:

Temperature	98.6°F
Blood pressure	120/75 mmHg
Heart rate	86 beats per minute
Respiratory rate	12 breaths per minute

Examinee's Tasks

1. Obtain a focused and relevant history.
2. Perform a focused and relevant physical examination.
3. Discuss your initial diagnostic impressions with the patient.
4. Discuss follow-up tests with the patient.

MY CHECKLIST

History of Present Illness. The Examinee:

1. _____
   _____
2. _____
3. _____
4. _____
5. _____
6. _____
7. _____
8. _____
   _____
9. _____
10. _____
11. _____
12. _____
13. _____
14. _____

Physical Examination. The Examinee:

15. _____
16. _____
17. _____
18. _____
19. _____
20. _____

Communication Skills. The Examinee:

21. _____
22. _____
23. _____
24. _____
25. _____

SP CHECKLIST FOR MS. OGELSBY

History of Present Illness. The Examinee:

___ 1. asked about the location of the pain ("It hurts in the front of my knee and it goes through to the back of my knee.")

___ 2. asked what I was doing at the time the pain began ("I was just playing the slot machine; I was sitting down.")

___ 3. asked if there was any recent trauma to the knee("No.")

___ 4. asked if I ever had a knee or joint swelling problem before ("No, could this be the beginning of arthritis?")

___ 5. asked what aggravates the pain ("It's worse with movement or anything touching the knee.")

___ 6. asked about any swelling ("Yes, it was swollen until the hotel doctor drained it; it was also red and warm.")

___ 7. asked if I had any past medical illnesses ("Yes, I have high blood pressure.")

___ 8. asked if I take any medications ("Only the pain pills the doctor gave me in Atlantic City and hydrochloro-thiazide 25 mg/day for my high blood pressure.")

___ 9. asked about any rashes ("No.")

___10. asked about fever ("No fever that I know of.")

___11. asked about alcohol use ("I did drink a few margaritas in the casino that day but that's very rare for me.")

___12. asked about tobacco use ("No.")

___13. asked about sexual history ("I'm married for 40 years to my husband.")

___14. asked about diet ("I eat mostly shellfish and potatoes.")

Physical Examination. The Examinee:

___15. checked my knee for a full range of motion (range of motion is decreased due to pain).

___16. checked for a knee effusion by the bulge or ballottement method (no effusion).

___17. palpated knee for tenderness (knee is tender).

___18. checked at least two other joints, i.e., hands, ankle, foot (other joints are normal).

___19. examined the other knee for comparison (normal right knee).

___20. asked me to walk around room (walks with noticeable limp).

Communication Skills. The Examinee:

___21. discussed the diagnostic possibilities with me (i.e., infectious arthritis, gout, pseudogout, bursitis).

___22. discussed the plan (blood work, urinalysis).

___23. explained the physical examination to me as it was being done.

___24. used language that I could understand.

___25. was empathetic.

If you performed 18 of these 25 tasks, you passed this test station.

You Have 10 Minutes to Complete Your Patient Note

HISTORY—Include significant positives and negatives from the history of present illness, past medical history, review of systems, and social and family history.

_____

_____

_____

_____

_____

_____

_____

_____

_____

_____

_____

PHYSICAL EXAMINATION—Indicate only the pertinent positive and negative findings related to the patient's chief complaint.

_____

_____

_____

_____

_____

_____

_____

_____

_____

_____

DIFFERENTIAL DIAGNOSIS—In order of likelihood, write no more than five differential diagnoses for this patient's current problems.

1. _____

2. _____

3. _____

4. _____

5. _____

DIAGNOSTIC WORKUP—Immediate plans for no more than five diagnostic studies.

1. _____

2. _____

3. _____

4. _____

5. _____

A SATISFACTORY PATIENT NOTE

HISTORY—Include significant positives and negatives from the history of present illness, past medical history, review of systems, and social and family history.

Mrs. Olympia Ogelsby is a 68-year-old woman who presents with left knee pain and swelling, which has been present for 2 days. The pain is associated with knee warmth, erythema, and tenderness. The pain started at rest; she denies trauma to the knee. The pain is located anteriorly and radiates posteriorly. Any movement or touching of the knee worsens the pain. Two days ago, a previous physician drained the knee and gave her some pills. The pills alleviate the pain. The patient denies any rashes, fever, or previous history of joint problems. She has a past medical history significant for hypertension controlled on HCTZ 25 mg daily. She did consume alcohol while on vacation but this is not a daily occurrence. She does not smoke cigarettes. She is sexually active only with her husband of 40 years. Her diet consists of shellfish and potatoes.

PHYSICAL EXAMINATION—Indicate only the pertinent positive and negative findings related to the patient's chief complaint.

T=98.6°F. BP=120/75 mmHg. HR=86 beats/min. RR=12 breaths/min. The patient appears her stated age of 68 years. She walks with a painful expression and a noticeable limp.
Skin: No rashes. No nodules or tophi visible.
Heart: Normal S_1 and S_2.
Lungs: Clear to auscultation.
Extremities: Left knee is erythematous, warm, and tender to palpation. ROM is limited due to pain. Negative bulge and ballottement signs. All other joints are normal.

DIFFERENTIAL DIAGNOSIS
In order of likelihood, write no more than five differential diagnoses for this patient's current problems.

1. gout

2. infectious arthritis

3. pseudogout

4. bursitis

5. cellulitis

DIAGNOSTIC WORKUP
Immediate plans for no more than five diagnostic studies.

1. CBC with differential

2. knee radiograph

3. electrolytes

4. uric acid level

5. BUN and creatinine

LEARNING OBJECTIVE FOR MRS. OGELSBY
RECOGNIZE THE COMMON ETIOLOGIES OF KNEE PAIN AND SWELLING
BASED ON HISTORY AND PHYSICAL EXAMINATION

Mrs. Olympia Ogelsby presents with left knee pain and swelling. The knee is warm, erythematous, and tender to palpation. She recently ingested alcohol, her diet is high in shellfish, and she takes hydro-chlorothiazide for hypertension. This history is consistent with gouty arthritis.

Gout is a metabolic disease associated with abnormal amounts of urates in the body and characterized by a monoarticular acute arthritis. Although the first metatarsal joint is the most susceptible joint, any joint may be affected. Although Mrs. Ogelsby was afebrile, fever is common. Tophi may be found in the external ears, hands, feet, olecranon, and prepatellar bursae. They are usually seen after several attacks of gout. Patients may have a leukocytosis and an elevated sedimentation rate. Radiographs are usually normal, but occasionally "rat-bite" punched out erosions are evident. Confirmation of gout is obtained by identifying the uric acid crystals by polarized examination of wet smears prepared from joint fluid aspiration. Nonsteroidal anti-inflammatory drugs (NSAIDs) have become the treatment of choice for patients with gout. Patients must be counseled on avoiding alcohol and foods high in purine. Medications, such as HCTZ and loop diuretics, inhibit renal excretion of uric acid and should be avoided.

Physical Examination Pearl: You should be familiar with the two methods of evaluating the knee for effusion. The "bulge" sign appears when you milk the medial knee upward and then tap the lateral knee. You will see the bulge of fluid return medially. The ballottement sign occurs when you apply downward pressure on the suprapatellar pouch and then push the patella downward toward the femur. When you release the patella, it will float or spring back upward.

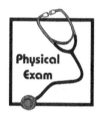

Patient Note Pearl: The **differential diagnosis** for knee pain in this patient includes infectious arthritis, gout, cellulitis, pseudogout, and bursitis. The **diagnostic workup** may include a CBC, electrolytes, BUN, creatinine, serum uric acid level, urinalysis, sedimentation rate, and a plain radiograph. Other patients with knee pain may warrant an arthritis screen (antinuclear antibodies, rheumatoid factor), Lyme titers, arthrocentesis, and an MRI scan if indicated.

Case 52

A 38-year-old man, Brian Beasley, presents to the emergency room complaining of anxiety. The triage nurse reports that the patient has a past history significant for psychiatric problems and that he has taken antipsychotic medications in the past. The patient is asking for help and more medication.

Vital Signs:

Temperature	99.0°F
Blood pressure	130/80 mmHg
Heart rate	90 beats per minute
Respiratory rate	14 breaths per minute

Examinee's Tasks

1. Obtain a focused and relevant history.
2. Obtain a mental status assessment.

MY CHECKLIST

History of Present Illness. The Examinee:

1. _____
2. _____
   _____
3. _____
4. _____
5. _____
   _____
6. _____
7. _____
8. _____
   _____
9. _____
   _____
10. _____
11. _____
12. _____
    _____
13. _____
14. _____
15. _____

Mental Status Examination. The Examinee:

16. _____
17. _____
18. _____
19. _____
20. _____
    _____
21. _____
22. _____
23. _____
24. _____
25. _____
26. _____
27. _____

28. _____

29. _____

30. _____

_____

31. _____

32. _____

33. _____

34. _____

35. _____

36. _____

37. _____

38. _____

_____

SP CHECKLIST FOR BRIAN BEASLEY

History of Present Illness. The Examinee:

____ 1. asked about the onset of the anxiety ("It started about 3 weeks ago.")

____ 2. asked about the duration of the anxiety ("It's constant; I can't even sleep due to the anxiety. Can you give me some medication?")

____ 3. asked about history of psychiatric disease ("Doctors say I have schizophrenia.")

____ 4. asked when the psychiatric problems started ("During college; I was prelaw when I started hearing voices.")

____ 5. asked about medications ("None right now. I've taken Haldol before but not for a year; I stopped them on my own.")

____ 6. asked about the last time I saw a psychiatrist ("A year ago.")

____ 7. asked about psychiatric admissions ("Five admissions over the last 15 years; the last one was 2 years ago.")

____ 8. asked about symptoms when he was hospitalized in the past ("I felt like I was being controlled and that people were plotting against me.")

____ 9. asked me to elaborate more about the plot ("People are checking my mail and following me; they are the ones responsible for my not getting a job.")

___10. asked where I was living ("I live with my mother; she is nagging me to get a job.")

___11. asked about friends ("None really.")

___12. asked about employment ("No one wants to hire me; I haven't worked in 2 years. It's not my fault though; it's a plot. The people checking my mail are out there saying that I'm a loser.")

___13. asked about tobacco use ("I've smoked 2 packs a day for 25 years.")

___14. asked about alcohol ("I drink 2 beers every day.")

___15. asked about illicit drug use ("Marijuana now and then.")

Mental Status Examination. The Examinee:

___16. checked my orientation to person, place and time (oriented to person, place, and time).

___17. asked about auditory hallucinations (none).

___18. asked about visual hallucinations (none).

___19. asked about olfactory hallucinations (none).

___20. asked about illusions or seeing things differently than they are, e.g., like a bush becomes a man at dusk ("No").

___21. checked my immediate memory, i.e., repeat numbers/objects (normal).

___22. checked my short-term memory, i.e., repeat items in 5 minutes (normal).

___23. checked my recent memory, i.e., weather yesterday (normal).

___24. checked my remote memory, i.e., birthday, social security number (normal).

___25. checked my insight into problems, i.e., do you need help? (patient admits that he needs help).

___26. checked my attention and concentration, i.e., serial sevens or spelling backwards (normal).

___27. checked my judgment, i.e., what would you do if you saw a fire in a wastebasket or found an envelope with a stamp and address on it? (normal).

___28. checked my abstract reasoning, i.e., proverbs or similarity/differences (normal).

___29. checked my fund of knowledge, i.e., presidents or months ("I'm a college graduate with a degree in political science; I would have been a trial lawyer if I had been able to get it together to apply to law school.")

___30. checked my ability to name objects, i.e., pen (normal).

___31. checked my ability to follow commands (normal).

___32. checked my left/right orientation (normal).

___33. checked my writing and visual spatial ability (normal).

___34. checked my drawing ability, i.e., clock (normal).

___35. asked about suicidal ideation (none).

___36. asked about a suicidal plan (none).

___37. asked about homicidal ideation (none).

___38. asked about paranoid ideation ("I do feel a little on edge; like something bad is going to happen. There is a plot out there against me. That's why I need medication again.")

If you performed 27 of these 38 tasks, you passed this test station.

You Have 10 Minutes to Complete Your Patient Note

HISTORY—Include significant positives and negatives from the history of present illness, past medical history, review of systems, and social and family history.

_____

_____

_____

_____

_____

_____

_____

_____

_____

_____

PHYSICAL EXAMINATION—Indicate only the pertinent positive and negative findings related to the patient's chief complaint.

_____

_____

_____

_____

_____

_____

_____

_____

_____

DIFFERENTIAL DIAGNOSIS—In order of likelihood, write no more than five differential diagnoses for this patient's current problems.

1. _____

2. _____

3. _____

4. _____

5. _____

DIAGNOSTIC WORKUP—Immediate plans for no more than five diagnostic studies.

1. _____

2. _____

3. _____

4. _____

5. _____

A SATISFACTORY PATIENT NOTE

HISTORY—Include significant positives and negatives from the history of present illness, past medical history, review of systems, and social and family history.

Mr. Brian Beasley is a 38-year-old man with a 15-year history of psychiatric problems. He has had five previous psychiatric hospitalizations, the most recent being 2 years ago. He has been prescribed Haldol but for 1 year has been noncompliant with his medication and psychiatric appointments. He is now presenting to the emergency room asking for help and requesting a prescription for Haldol. He is feeling anxious and is having difficulty sleeping. Mr. Beasley has been unemployed for 2 years and is living with his mother, who is nagging him to get a job. He is not having hallucinations or illusions but does think that people are plotting against him and are trying to control him. He feels that it these people who are responsible for his inability to get a job; they are checking his mail and telling future employers that he is a loser and shouldn't be hired. He has smoked 2 packs of cigarettes per day for 25 years and drinks 2 beers daily. He occasionally uses marijuana. He has no friends or support system other than his mother. His psychiatric problems started while he was a college student majoring in Political Science. He was able to graduate but was never able to "get it together" to apply to law school. It was his dream to become a trial lawyer.

PHYSICAL EXAMINATION—Indicate only the pertinent positive and negative findings related to the patient's chief complaint.

T=99.0°F. BP=130/80 mmHg. HR=90 beats/min. RR=14 breaths/min. The patient is casually dressed in jeans and sneakers. He has good eye contact and is responsive to questions. He is neat and clean. He is polite, intelligent, and articulate. He becomes restless and fidgety when asked sensitive questions.

Mental Status Examination: Alert and 0×3.

No auditory, visual, or olfactory hallucinations.

Immediate memory: Normal.

Short-term memory: Normal.

Recent memory: Normal.

Remote memory: Normal.

Insight into problem: Good insight.

Attention and concentration: Good.

Judgment: Good.

Abstract reasoning: Normal.

Fund of knowledge: Intelligent.

Naming objects: Normal.
Follows commands: Normal.
Right/left orientation: Normal.
Writing/visuospatial ability: Normal.
Drawing ability: Normal.
Suicidal ideation: None.
Suicidal plan: None.
Homicidal ideation: None.
Delusions: Yes.
Illusions: None.
Paranoid ideation: Yes.

DIFFERENTIAL DIAGNOSIS	DIAGNOSTIC WORKUP
In order of likelihood, write no more than five differential diagnoses for this patient's current problems.	Immediate plans for no more than five diagnostic studies.
1. schizophrenia	1. obtain old medical records
2. paranoid ideation	2. counseling
3.	3.
4.	4.
5.	5.

LEARNING OBJECTIVE FOR BRIAN BEASLEY
PERFORM A MENTAL STATUS EXAMINATION IN A PATIENT WITH A PSYCHIATRIC ILLNESS

The schizophrenic disorders are manifest by disruption of thinking, mood, and overall behavior as well as difficulty filtering external stimuli. Mr. Beasley is not experiencing any hallucinations and has no illusions or homicidal/suicidal ideation (standard questions that are posed to a standardized patient with a psychiatric problem), but he does feel as if people were controlling him and plotting against him. He has delusions (beliefs not based on truth) and is paranoid with an impaired thought process. Step 2 CS examinees must be thorough and patient in performing the mental status examination. Often only one or two of the categories will be abnormal.

Patient Note Pearl: The **differential diagnosis** for Brian Beasley is schizophrenia and paranoid ideation. The **workup** includes the need to obtain the patient's old medical records and to begin counseling.

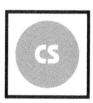

Case 53

A 44-year-old woman named Margaret Neutron presents to your office complaining of weight loss.

Vital Signs:

Temperature	98.6°F
Blood pressure	130/80 mmHg
Heart rate	100 beats per minute
Respiratory rate	14 breaths per minute

Examinee's Tasks

1. Obtain a focused and relevant history.
2. Perform a focused and relevant physical examination.
3. Discuss your initial diagnostic impressions with the patient.
4. Discuss follow-up tests with the patient.

MY CHECKLIST

History of Present Illness. The Examinee:

1. _____
2. _____
3. _____
4. _____
   _____
5. _____
6. _____
7. _____
8. _____
9. _____
10. _____
11. _____
12. _____
13. _____
14. _____
15. _____

Physical Examination. The Examinee:

16. _____
17. _____
18. _____
19. _____
20. _____
21. _____
22. _____
23. _____
24. _____
25. _____
26. _____
27. _____

Communication Skills. The Examinee:

28. _____
29. _____
30. _____
31. _____
32. _____

SP CHECKLIST FOR MS. NEUTRON

History of Present Illness. The Examinee:

___ 1.   asked about amount of weight loss ("Ten pounds.")

___ 2.   asked over what period of time the weight loss occurred ("It's only been happening over the last month.")

___ 3.   asked about appetite ("My appetite is great; I'm eating fine.")

___ 4.   asked about insomnia ("Yes, I can't go to sleep at night until 2 in the morning; that's never happened to me before.")

___ 5.   asked about fatigue ("Yes, I'm tired all the time.")

___ 6.   asked about weakness ("Yes, my legs feel weak lately, especially when I have to climb stairs.")

___ 7.   asked about any heat intolerance ("Yes, I'm always hot and sweaty.")

___ 8.   asked about gastrointestinal symptoms ("I have a lot of diarrhea lately; five bowel movements per day.")

___ 9.   asked about palpitations ("Yes, I have palpitations.")

___10.   asked about tremors ("Yes, my hands are always shaking lately; it's like I'm on edge and tense all the time.")

___11.   asked if I had any past medical illnesses ("No.")

___12.   asked if I take any medications ("No.")

___13.   asked about alcohol use ("None.")

___14.   asked about tobacco use ("No.")

___15.   asked about family history ("My mother has a low thyroid; do you think that's what I have?")

Physical Examination. The Examinee:

___16.   checked my pulse (tachycardia).

___17.   checked for tremors by asking me to stretch out my hands (fine tremors present).

___18.   palpated my thyroid gland (normal nontender thyroid).

___19.   asked me to swallow to check my thyroid gland (gland moves with swallowing).

___20.   checked my eye movements (EOMI).

___21.   checked my lungs in four places (normal lung examination).

___22.   checked my heart (normal heart examination).

___23.   checked my upper leg strength (decreased strength).

___24.   checked my lower leg strength (normal strength).

___25.   checked arm strength (normal).

___26.   Checked reflexes at knee (increased reflexes).

___27.   Checked arm reflexes (increased reflexes).

Communication Skills. The Examinee:

___28.   discussed the diagnostic possibilities with me (i.e., hyperthyroidism or anxiety).

___29.   discussed the plan (blood work, thyroid hormone levels).

___30.   explained the physical examination to me as it was being done.

___31.   used language that I could understand.

___32.   was empathetic.

If you performed 23 of these 32 tasks, you passed this test station.

You Have 10 Minutes to Complete Your Patient Note

HISTORY—Include significant positives and negatives from the history of present illness, past medical history, review of systems, and social and family history.

_____

_____

_____

_____

_____

_____

_____

_____

_____

_____

PHYSICAL EXAMINATION—Indicate only the pertinent positive and negative findings related to the patient's chief complaint.

_____

_____

_____

_____

_____

_____

_____

_____

_____

_____

DIFFERENTIAL DIAGNOSIS—In order of likelihood, write no more than five differential diagnoses for this patient's current problems.

1. _____

2. _____

3. _____

4. _____

5. _____

DIAGNOSTIC WORKUP—Immediate plans for no more than five diagnostic studies.

1. _____

2. _____

3. _____

4. _____

5. _____

A SATISFACTORY PATIENT NOTE

HISTORY—Include significant positives and negatives from the history of present illness, past medical history, review of systems, and social and family history.

Ms. Margaret Neutron is a 44-year-old woman who presents with the chief complaint of weight loss. Over the last month, she has lost 10 pounds despite an increase in appetite. She is feeling tense and anxious and has noticed that her hands are tremulous. She is always fatigued and has difficulty falling asleep; she is often awake until 2 in the morning. Ms. Neutron feels that her legs are weak, especially when climbing stairs. She also admits to diarrhea, heat intolerance, and palpitations. She has never been ill before and takes no medications. She does not smoke cigarettes, drink alcohol, or use illicit drugs. Family history is positive for her mother having hypothyroidism.

PHYSICAL EXAMINATION—Indicate only the pertinent positive and negative findings related to the patient's chief complaint.

T=98.6°F. BP=130/80 mmHg. HR=100 beats/min. RR=14 breaths/min. The patient is a restless and anxious woman who appears her stated age.

Skin: Moist and warm. Hair fine.

HEENT: PERLA. EOMI. No lid lag. +Stare.

Thyroid gland not palpable. No bruits.

Heart: Tachycardia. Regular rhythm. Normal S_1 and S_2.

Lungs: Clear to auscultation.

Abdomen: Normal BS. Nontender.

Extremities: Fine tremors with hands outstretched.

Neurologic: Alert and oriented×3.

Strength UE proximal and distal muscles 5/5.

Strength LE proximal muscles 4/5.

Strength LE distal muscles 5/5.

DTR 3+ diffusely.

DIFFERENTIAL DIAGNOSIS
In order of likelihood, write no more than 5 differential diagnoses for this patient's current problems.

1. hyperthyroidism
2. anxiety
3. mania
4.
5.

DIAGNOSTIC WORKUP
Immediate plans for no more than five diagnostic studies.

1. CBC
2. electrolytes
3. TSH and free T4 levels
4. antimicrosomal antibodies
5. T3

LEARNING OBJECTIVE FOR MS. NEUTRON
RECOGNIZE HYPERTHYROIDISM IN THE PATIENT
PRESENTING WITH WEIGHT LOSS

Patients with hyperthyroidism may complain of restlessness, anxiety, heat intolerance, increased sweating, palpitations, fatigue, muscle cramps, diarrhea, and weight loss. Ophthalmopathy may occur in 20 to 40 percent of patients and usually consists of chemosis, conjunctivitis, and mild proptosis. Other physical examination findings may include stare and lid lag. Patients may have hyperreflexia and proximal muscle weakness.

Patient Note Pearl: The **differential diagnosis** for weight loss includes hyperthyroidism, anxiety neurosis, and mania. **Workup** may include TSH, free T4 and T3 (RIA) levels. A ^{123}I uptake scan, and antibodies (antithyroglobulin and antimicrosomal) may also be indicated.

The Common Encounters for Each Specialty

Common Encounters in Family Medicine

Abdominal pain
Acute pericarditis
Adult health maintenance
Advance directives
Ambulatory management of HIV
Anemia
Anxiety
Assessment of functional health status in the elderly
Asthma
Behavioral disturbances
Care for common injuries (burns, bites, cuts)
Care of the newborn
Caring for the dying
Caring for the elderly
Cerebrovascular disease
Chest pain
Chronic obstructive pulmonary disease
Compliance with medication regimen
Congestive heart failure
Conjunctivitis
Contraception/safe sex counseling
Dizziness
Dementia
Depression
Dermatologic problems
Diabetes mellitus
Diarrhea
Elder abuse
Ethical issues in primary care
Exercise prescriptions
Family structure/family counseling
Fatigue
Fever
Growth and development of children
Headache
Heart disease
HIV testing and counseling
Home care and utilization of community resources
Hypertension
Low back pain
Marriage counseling
Menstrual irregularities
Musculoskeletal injuries
Nutrition prescriptions
Obesity
Occupational medicine
Office gynecology
Otitis
Peripheral vascular disease
Pharyngitis/sinusitis
Pneumonia
Post–myocardial infarction rehabilitation

Prenatal examination
Preventive cardiology
Seizure
Sexual abuse/assault
Smoking cessation and guidance
Somatization disorder
Stress management
Substance abuse
Suturing/minor surgery
Urinary tract infection
Vertigo
Well-baby care/well-child care

Common Encounters in Internal Medicine
Abdominal pain
Advance directives
Anemia
Back pain
Chest pain
Claudication
Confusion
Constipation
Cough
Diarrhea
Dizziness
Fatigue
Fever
Headache
Hearing loss
Hematemesis
Hematuria
Hemoptysis
HIV counseling and care
Impotence
"I need a physical exam."
"I need my blood pressure checked."
"I need my sugar checked."
"I passed out." (syncope)
Jaundice
Joint pain
Leg swelling (edema)
Lymphadenopathy
Melena
Painful urination (dysuria)
Palpitations
Rash
Rectal bleeding (hematochezia)
Shortness of breath (dyspnea)
Sore throat
Swollen thyroid
Tremors
Vertigo
Vision loss
Vomiting
Weakness
Weight loss

Common Encounters in Obstetrics and Gynecology

Abnormal Pap smear
Abnormal uterine bleeding
Adnexal mass
Amenorrhea
Breast mass/breast disease
Calculation of gestational age and estimated date of confinement
Cancer screening
Chronic pelvic pain
Common complaints during pregnancy
Contraception and family planning
Detection of high-risk pregnancy
Detection of medical or surgical conditions that may complicate pregnancy
Disorders of lactation
Domestic violence
Drug, tobacco, and alcohol use in pregnancy
Dysmenorrhea
Dyspareunia
Ectopic pregnancy
Endometrial biopsy
Endometriosis
Fibroid uterus
First-trimester bleeding
Genetic counseling
Hirsutism
Infertility
Menopause
Miscarriage/spontaneous abortion
Normal pregnancy
Nutritional counseling in pregnancy
Pelvic inflammatory disease
Placenta previa
Postmenopausal bleeding
Postpartum care
Premenstrual syndrome
Prenatal care
Sexual assault and abuse
Sexual dysfunction
Sexually transmitted disease
Urinary tract infection
Vaginal discharge
Vaginitis
Voluntary termination of pregnancy/induced abortion

Common Encounters in Pediatrics

Abdominal pain
Adolescent high-risk sexual behavior
Anemia
Breast feeding
Child abuse
Congenital heart disease
Cough
Cystic fibrosis
Dehydration
Developmental evaluation
Diarrhea/gastroenteritis

Earache/otitis media
Hearing loss
Hematologic malignancies
Hematuria
Infants with feeding problems
Infections in children
Joint pain
Language developmental problems
Nutrition guidelines and obesity
Orthopedic evaluation in a child
Age-appropriate physical examination
Poisoning and ingestions
Proteinuria

Common Encounters in Psychiatry
Alcohol-related disorders
Anorexia, bulimia
Bipolar disorder
Complications of psychiatric drugs
Delirium
Delusional or paranoid disorders
Dementia
Depression
Dissociative disorders
Normal grief
Obsessive-compulsive disorder
Panic disorder and phobias
Personality disorders
Posttraumatic stress disorder
Schizophrenia
Sexual disorders (erectile disorder)
Somatoform disorders
Stress reduction and management
Substance abuse
Suicidal patient

Common Encounters in Surgery
Abdominal mass
Acute abdominal pain
Breast mass
Burns
Electrolyte abnormalities in a post-op patient
Epistaxis
Gastrointestinal cancers
Head trauma evaluation
Hernia
Infections (e.g., cellulitis, diverticulitis)
Intestinal obstruction
Kidney stone
Multiple injury trauma evaluation
Postoperative fever
Postoperative shock
Vascular emergencies/use of Doppler ultrasound

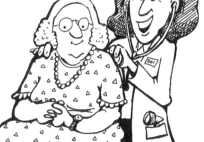

Medicine

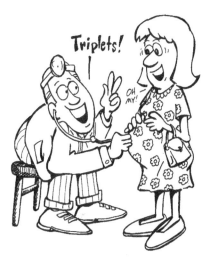

Obstetrics & Gynecology

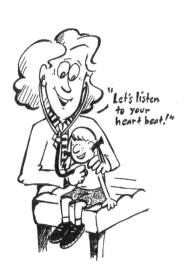

Pediatrics

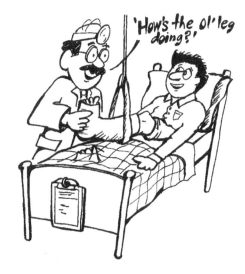

Surgery

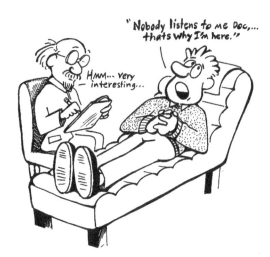

Psychiatry

Section D: Communication Skills : Decreasing Your Chances of Failing

Improving Your Communication Skills Quickly

■ The ECFMG has tested approximately 2000 candidates from July 1, 1998, through January 31, 2004, using the Clinical Skills Assessment (CSA), which is the precursor to the Step 2 CS (Clinical Skills Examination).

- 82 percent of candidates successfully passed the CSA.
- 80 percent of those who failed the CSA did so in the patient–doctor communication (COM) section.

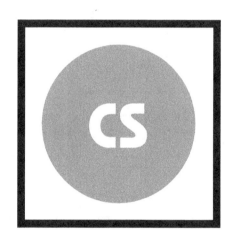

Following are 15 effective strategies to improve your communication skills and decrease your chances of failing the CSA:

1. Introduce yourself to the patient. Politely confirm the patient's name.

2. Empathize. Show genuine concern for the patient.

3. Acknowledge everything the patient says or does that is unusual.

4. A positive response to a question from the patient must be followed up by the examinee with a statement or question (e.g., "What color was the loose stool?" "Could you describe the chest pain?" "How did that make you feel?" "Tell me more about that.").

5. Make sure that your mood and body language are appropriate.

6. Wash your hands before touching the patient.

7. Warm your hands and stethoscope before touching the patient.

8. Keep the patient comfortable at all times.

9. The patient will disrobe if you request this, but try to keep the patient draped. Respect the patient's privacy and modesty. Do not examine through the gown.

10. Do not attempt to perform a rectal exam, pelvic exam, genital exam, or breast exam (they can be included in the *patient note,* however, if relevant).

11. Answer all patient questions. Always give the patient differential diagnoses (at least three) and explain your diagnostic plans. Never restrict yourself to a single diagnosis.

12. Be clear when asking questions or giving information; use medical language appropriately. Explain all medical terms.

13. Don't be afraid to obtain a drug, alcohol, tobacco, or sexual history if relevant. Don't shy away from giving advice on sexual matters if they are brought up by the patient. Be thorough.

14. Be sincere, direct, and honest. When you do not know something, say so.

15. Remain confident and calm.

The Day of the Step 2 CS

<u>**8:30 A.M.**</u>

■ Step 2 CS orientation starts

■ Emphasis on the rules of the patient encounter:

–There are no children presenting as SPs. There are, however, caregivers for children and elderly patients.

–Some stations may be telephone interviews.

–Corneal, rectal, pelvic, genitourinary, and female breast examinations are not permitted.

–You may take notes (remember to maintain eye contact with the patient while taking notes).

–The *patient note* should *not* include treatment, hospitalizations, referrals, or consultations.

–An announcement will tell you when to begin the encounter, when there are 5 minutes left, and when the encounter is completed.

–If you finish early, you may leave the examination room but you may not then reenter it.

■ Demonstration of the diagnostic instruments to be used for the actual patient encounters:

–Instructions on how to use an ophthalmoscope/otoscope.

–How to use the examination table extension.

–You are expected to bring your own stethoscope and white lab coat.

■ The Step 2 CS lasts for about 8 hours. There are two breaks (30 minutes after case 4 for lunch and 15 minutes after case 7). You are not allowed to leave a patient encounter to use the restroom.

<u>**9:30 A.M.**</u>

■ The patient encounters begin.

The Top Ten Causes of CS Examination Failure

1. *Interrupting* the patient or *rushing* the patient's responses. *Cutting off* the patient's response to pose another question.

2. Failing to use the examination table extension when the patient is reclined (*do not* let the patient's legs dangle).

3. Running out of time and leaving the room improperly. *Do not run out.* Attempt closure, say good-bye, and tell the patient that you will be back.

4. *Attempting* to perform a corneal, pelvic, rectal, breast, or genitourinary exam. Include it in the workup plan *after* you inform the patient that you plan to do the exam.

5. *Using technical terminology* or medical jargon. Not giving clear explanations. Explaining tests and findings in terms not understandable to the patient.

6. *Not talking to the patient* as you are examining him or her and not explaining *what* you are doing and *why* you are doing it. *Not letting the patient know* when you are beginning the physical examination.

7. Writing a patient note in an *illogical sequence.* Failing to group similar data together in the patient note.

8. Writing *illegibly* (*do not* write outside the margins, since the computer will not pick up this information when the patient note is scanned).

9. *Omitting critical elements* in the patient note. Failing to include pertinent negatives and positives. Failing to portray the patient's problem accurately. Writing a patient note that lacks accuracy and specificity.

10. *Giving the patient a premature diagnosis instead of differential diagnoses.*

The Final Preparation: A Review of the Common Step 2 CS Scenarios

It is impossible to list every Step 2 CS case you might encounter, since new cases are being written on a daily basis. The cases below, however, are commonly tested scenarios.

Chest Pain Scenarios

1. **Chest pressure in a 45-year-old female.**
   HPI: lasts for 1 to 2 minutes, radiating to the jaw.
   Aggravated by exertion, relieved by rest and nitroglycerin.
   Think: Angina Pectoris, Myocardial Ischemia

2. **Burning chest pain in a 29-year-old male.**
   HPI: Pain lasts for hours, relieved by antacids.
   Think: GERD, PUD

3. **Sharp, stabbing chest pain in a 30-year-old female.**
   HPI: Aggravated by stress and deep breathing.
   Pain relieved by ASA.
   PE: (+) Chest wall tenderness.
   Think: Costochondritis or Tietze's Syndrome

4. **Sharp right-sided chest pain.**
   HPI: Worse lying down and improved when sitting up.
   Think: Pericarditis

5. **Chest discomfort for 3 months.**
   HPI: Brought on by exertion and cold weather; has abstained from sex with his wife due to fear of having pain.
   PE: stoic man who displays no emotion
   Think: Coronary Artery Disease, Acute Coronary Syndrome, Angina

6. **Abrupt onset of right-sided chest pain.**
   HPI: (+) SOB. Pain is sharp and severe.
   PE: Shallow breathing, splinting, diminished breath sounds on right side.
   Think: Pneumothorax

7. **Abrupt onset of right-sided chest pain.**
   HPI: (+) SOB. Pain is pleuritic in nature. Recent travel.
   PE: Tachypnea, red, warm, and tender extremity.
   Think: Pulmonary Embolus, Pulmonary Infarction

8. **Progressively worsening diffuse chest pain.**
   HPI: (+) SOB. (+) cough. Pain is pleuritic in nature.
   PMH: Sickle Cell Disease
   Think: Sickle Cell Crises, Acute Chest Syndrome

Women Health Scenarios

1. **A 38-year-old female brought to the ER by her husband.**
   HPI: Has multiple facial and body injuries.
   PMH: Third hospitalization for the same problem.
   PE: BP: 100/60 mmHg. PR: 78 beats/min. RR: 22 breaths/ min. Temp: 99.8°F.
   Think: Domestic Violence

2. **A 17-year-old female brought by sister for contraceptive counseling.**
   HPI: Patient is 6 weeks postpartum. Boyfriend does not like condoms. Boyfriend has three other children. Patient thinks that birth control pills make you fat.
   Think: Parenting classes, counsel to finish high school, possible abusive relationship with boyfriend, ask to meet boyfriend and educate patient regarding contraception options.

3. **A 31-year-old female with frothy gray vaginal discharge.**
   HPI: Vaginal discharge described as having a fishy odor.
   Think: Bacterial Vaginosis

4. **A 25-year-old college student with green-yellow discharge.**
   HPI: Vaginal discharge is frothy and malodorous.
   Social history: Sexually active.
   Think: Trichomonas Vaginalis

5. **A 39-year-old female with vaginal discharge.**
   HPI: Discharge is white and curdy. Patient has diabetes.
   Think: *Candida albicans*

6. **A 41-year-old with vaginal bleeding.**
   HPI: Postcoital bleeding and metrorrhagia.
   Think: Cervical Cancer

7. **A 65-year-old nulliparous female with vaginal bleeding.**
   HPI: Postmenopausal female with abdominal pain.
   Think: Endometrial Cancer

8. **A 28-year-old woman worried about a change in her periods.**
   HPI: Has no periods for 3 months. (+) Galactorrhea
   PE: No masculinization signs. No visual field cuts.
   Pelvic examination report states "no ovaries palpated"
   Think: Pregnancy, Polycystic Ovary Disease, Prolactinoma, Adrenal Tumor or Thyroid Disease

Joint Problem Scenarios

1. **A 56-year-old female complaining of knee pain.**
   Family History: Her mother had rheumatoid arthritis.
   PE: Temp: 102.5°F. Redness and swelling over knee, multiple joints involved.
   Think: Rheumatoid Arthritis

2. **Knee pain in a sexually active female.**
   HPI: Sexually promiscuous. Does not use protection.
   PE: Febrile. Swollen, tender, and warm knee. (+) Skin lesions.
   Think: Septic Arthritis, Disseminated Gonococcal Infection

3. **A 49-year-old man with shoulder pain.**
   HPI: Diet high in meats. (+) Alcohol use. No trauma.
   PMH: Swollen toe 4 years ago.
   PE: Tender and warm shoulder. Decreased range of motion.
   Think: Gout

4. **A 22-year-old gymnast with recent knee trauma.**
   HPI: Twisted her knee during floor exercises.
   PE: Tender and warm knee. (+) Anterior draw test. (+) Lachman maneuver. (+) Bulge sign. (+) Ballottement sign
   Think: Anterior Cruciate Ligament Injury

5. **A 26-year-old with bilateral knee pain.**
   HPI: No history of trauma.
   PMH: Sickle cell disease
   PE: All joints are tender and warm.
   Think: Sickle Cell Crises

6. **A 70-year-old woman presents with bilateral knee pain.**
   HPI: Has history of osteoarthritis. Knee pain has been worsening. Has been taking her prescription for NSAID.
   PE: Knee joints are swollen and warm.
   Think: Osteoarthritis and Medication Failure

Gastrointestinal Scenarios

1. **Epigastric pain in a 36-year-old male.**
   HPI: Radiation to the back. (+) Nausea and vomiting, weakness.
   Social History: (+) ETOH abuse.
   Think: Acute Pancreatitis

2. **A 28-year-old male with vague abdominal pain.**
   HPI: Epigastric pain which later localizes to the right lower quadrant.
   PE: Low-grade fever. (+) Rebound tenderness and guarding.
   Think: Appendicitis

3. **A 32-year-old female with periumbilical pain for 3 months.**
   HPI: Abdominal pain worsened by stress, relieved by defecation. Not relieved by antacids. Pain never interferes with sleep. Episodes of diarrhea alternating with constipation. Abdominal distention noted.
   Think: Irritable Bowel Syndrome

4. **A 45-year-old obese female with severe RUQ abdominal pain.**
   HPI: Pain precipitated by fatty meals, nausea, and vomiting.
   PE: Tenderness on palpation (+) Murphy's sign.
   Think: Acute Cholecystitis

5. **A young woman with daily morning vomiting for 1 week.**
   HPI: Last menstrual period 10 weeks ago.
   Think: Hyperemesis Gravidarum

6. **A 72-year-old man with positive FOBT.**
   HPI: Progressive weight loss.
   FH: Father had colon cancer.
   Think: Colon Cancer

7. **A 33-year-old female with rectal bleeding.**
   HPI: (+) Diarrhea, rectal pain, and tenesmus.
   FH: Mother had colitis.
   Social History: Ex-smoker.
   Think: Inflammatory Bowel Disease

8. **A 61-year-old female with a chief complaint of diarrhea.**
   HPI: Hospitalized a week ago and was on antibiotics. Foul-smelling watery diarrhea with lower abdominal cramps.
   Think: *Clostridium difficile* (pseudomembranous) Colitis.

9. **An 18-year-old male with diarrhea.**
   HPI: (+) Recent travel to Mexico.
   PE: Tachycardia.
   Think: Traveler's Diarrhea

10. **A 25-year-old female with diarrhea.**
    HPI: Aggravated by milk, relieved by fasting.
    Episodes of abdominal cramps and bloating.
    Think: Lactose Intolerance or Malabsorption

11. **48-year-old woman with crampy abdominal pain and diarrhea.**
    HPI: Recent travel to Maine where she drank stream water.
    Has pet turtle.
    Think: *Giardia* or *Salmonella*

12. **A 39-year-old man vomiting blood.**
    HPI: (+) Retching. Takes aspirin daily. Passed black stool. Vague abdominal pain. Drinks alcohol and smokes cigarettes. Six cups of coffee per day.
    PE: Orthostasis is present. No stigmata of liver disease.
    Think: Mallory-Weiss Tear, Gastritis, Esophageal Varices, or PUD

13. **24-year-old man with watery diarrhea.**
    HPI: No travel history or history of contaminated food or water. Living with girlfriend but has had homosexual relationships in the past.
    Think: AIDS Diarrhea

Back Pain Scenarios

1. **A 52-year old-male complaining of back pain.**
   HPI: Sudden, severe chest pain with radiation to the back.
   PE: BP: 160/110 mmHg. BP varies in left and right arms.
   PMH: (+) Uncontrolled hypertension
   Think: Aortic Dissection

2. **A 60-year-old male truck driver with the sudden onset of low back pain.**
   PE: Pain radiates down the thighs and below the knee. Straight leg raise (SLR) maneuver positive.
   Think: Disc Herniation

3. **A 39-year-old male construction worker with low back pain.**
HPI: Pain is aggravated by heavy lifting. Relieved by rest.
PE: (+) Tenderness to palpation, (−) SLR maneuver
Think: Lumbosacral Sprain

4. **A 65-year-old obese male with worsening lower back pain.**
HPI: Back pain is precipitated by walking or prolonged standing, relieved by sitting. Pain worse walking downhill than uphill.
Think: Lumbar Stenosis

Psychiatric Scenarios

1. **A 29-year-old female complaining of constipation.**
HPI: Mother recently sent to a nursing home for Alzheimer's disease. Patient feeling very sad and guilty.
Think: Depression

2. **A 29-year-old woman with history of headaches.**
HPI: Headaches relieved by Valium. Patient wants refill. Patient is seductive and manipulative. Eventually becomes hostile. States she lost her last prescription. Has recently lost job.
Think: Benzodiazepine Dependence and Alcohol Abuse

3. **49-year-old mother of two grown children presents with fatigue.**
HPI: Drinks six glasses of wine daily. Slapped her daughter yesterday. Had recent minor car accident. Husband away on business trips often.
PE: (+) CAGE. Breath smells of mouthwash.
Think: Alcohol Abuse and Possible Depression

4. **A young woman with headaches.**
HPI: Has runny nose. Snorts cocaine with friends. Poor appetite. Ten pound weight loss. Has unprotected sex occasionally. Having financial problems. Now forging checks to buy cocaine.
PE: Nasal mucosa is red and inflamed. No perforation.
Think: Cocaine Addiction and STD Risk

Respiratory Scenarios

1. **A 32-year-old female complaining of shortness of breath.**
HPI: Acute onset of fever and productive cough.
PE: BP: 140/90 mmHg. PR: 115 beats/min. RR: 28 breaths/min. Temp: 103°F.
Think: Bacterial Pneumonia

2. **A 16-year-old complaining of the sudden onset of cough.**
   PMH: Recurrent attacks.
   PE: (+) Wheezing.
   Think: Bronchial Asthma

3. **A 72-year-old complaining of a chronic cough.**
   HPI: Cough is blood-streaked occasionally.
   Social Hx: Has smoked two packs of cigarettes per day for 50 years.
   ROS: (+) Weight loss, malaise.
   Think: Lung Cancer

Pediatric Scenarios

1. **A 7-month-old boy with diarrhea.**
   HPI: Mother is dressed sexily. Single mother. Has not kept past immunization appointments. Does not know how to mix formula. Mother has poor insight and judgment.
   PE: Growth chart shown to examinee reveals no growth since infant was 4 months old.
   Think: Failure to Thrive, Inadequate Caloric Intake

2. **A 4-year-old girl with a chief complaint of ear pain.**
   HPI: Always pulling and tugging at ear.
   PE: Febrile and irritable.
   Think: Otitis Media

3. **An 18-month-old boy with a chief complaint of vomiting.**
   HPI: Infant is picky eater. Does not like to chew meats. Drinks six 8-ounce bottles of milk daily. Was breast-fed for 1 month. Peeling paint in old house. Speech single words only. Brother also ill. (+) Pica likes to chew on paint chips and pillows.
   PE: Infant is pale and febrile.
   Think: Lead Poisoning or Iron Deficiency Anemia
   TIP: *Always instruct the mother/caretaker to bring the child to your office or to the emergency room for a complete examination.*

Other Very Common Scenarios

1. **A 61-year-old female complaining of fatigue.**
   HPI: The patient complains of repeated yawning all day, hoarseness, cold intolerance, and depression.
   PE: BP: 90/70 mmHg. PR: 50 beats/min. RR: 18 breaths/min. Temp: 96.4°F
   Think: Hypothyroidism

2. **A 26-year old female complaining of wrist pain.**
   HPI: (+) Hand tingling of first, second, and third digits.
   SH: Patient works as a secretary.
   PE: (+) Phalen's and Tinel's signs.
   Think: Carpal Tunnel Syndrome

3. **A 56-year-old male complaining of bloody urine.**
   Social History: (+) Tobacco for 40 years.
   PE: BP: 110/80 mmHg. PR: 85 beats/min. RR: 18 breaths/min. Temp: 100.2°F
      (+) Bitemporal wasting, (+) Flank pain.
   Think: Renal Cell Carcinoma

4. **A 26-year-old man with palpitations that resolved spontaneously.**
   HPI: Palpitations lasted 20 minutes. Has had several times before but never sought help. ECG given to examinee shows supraventricular tachycardia. Has fast-paced job. Drinks coffee. Smokes cigarettes. Drinks beer daily and more on weekends. No drug use. Recently divorced.
   PE: HR is 80 beats/min. BP 110/70 mmHg. Has fine tremors.
   Think: Anxiety, Hyperthyroidism or Alcohol-Related Heart Disease

5. **A 65-year-old woman with syncope.**
   HPI: Under financial pressure. Husband has abused her in the past. Children away at college. Has had two previous episodes. Before syncope, she becomes light-headed and develops paresthesias of her hands and periorbital areas. Hands become stiff.
   Think: Hyperventilation or Panic Disorder

6. **Diabetes Medication Refill**

7. **Asthma Medication Refill**

8. **Hypertension Medication Refill**

9. **Preemployment Checkup**

10. **Smoking Cessation Counseling**

11. **Terminal Cancer Counseling**

12. **HIV Counseling**

- Familiarize yourself with all of the above cases.

- Memorize the different scenarios for each symptom and use them to expand your differential diagnoses.

- Practice these cases and time yourself.

Appendix: Allowable Abbreviations for the Patient Note

Abd	abdomen
AIDS	acquired immune deficiency syndrome
AP	anteroposterior
BP	blood pressure
BUN	blood urea nitrogen
CABG	coronary artery bypass grafting
CBC	complete blood count
CCU	cardiac care unit
cig	cigarettes
CHF	congestive heart failure
C/O	complaining of
COPD	chronic obstructive pulmonary disease
CPR	cardiopulmonary resuscitation
CT	computed tomography
CVA	cerebrovascular accident
CVP	central venous pressure
CXR	chest x-ray
DM	diabetes mellitus
DTR	deep tendon reflexes
ECG	electrocardiogram
ED	emergency department
EMT	emergency medical technician
ENT	ears, nose, and throat
EOM	extraocular muscles
ETOH	alcohol
Ext	extremities
FH	family history
GI	gastrointestinal
GU	genitourinary
HEENT	head, eyes, ears, nose, and throat
HIV	human immunodeficiency virus
HR	heart rate
HTN	hypertension
hx	history
H/O	history of
IM	intramuscularly
IV	intravenously
JVD	jugular venous distention
KUB	kidney, ureter, and bladder
L	left

LMP	last menstrual period
LP	lumbar puncture
MI	myocardial infarction
MRI	magnetic resonance imaging
MVA	motor vehicle accident
Negative	(−)
Neuro	neurologic
NIDDM	non-insulin-dependent diabetes mellitus
NKA	no known allergies
NKDA	no known drug allergy
NL	normal limits
NSR	normal sinus rhythm
P	pulse
PA	posteroanterior
PERLA	pupils equal, react to light and accommodation
PO	orally
positive	(+)
PT	prothrombin time
PTT	partial prothrombin time
PUD	peptic ulcer disease
R	right
RR	respiratory rate
RBC	red blood cells
SH	social history
T	temperature
TIA	transient ischemic attack
U/A	urinalysis
URI	upper respiratory tract infection
WBC	white blood cells
WNL	within normal limits

Index of Practice Cases

OBSTETRICS AND GYNECOLOGY

PEDIATRICS

PSYCHIATRY

SURGERY

References

PRACTICE CASES

Physical Examination

Seidel, H. M., Ball, J. W., Dains, J. E., Benedict, G. W., Kissane, D. W. 2002. Mosby's Guide to Physical Examination, 5th ed. St. Louis, Missouri: Mosby.

Family Medicine

Sloane, P. D., Slatt, L. M., Curtis, P. 2002. Essentials of Family Medicine. 4th ed. Baltimore, Maryland: Lippincott Williams & Wilkins.

Medicine

Tierney, L. M., Jr., McPhee, S. J., Papadakis, M. A., eds. 2003. Current Medical Diagnosis and Treatment. 43rd ed. New York: McGraw-Hill.

Kasper, D. L., Braunwald, E., Fauci, A. S., Hauser, S. L., Longo, D. L., Jameson, J. L., eds. 2004. Harrison's Principles of Internal Medicine. 16th ed. New York: McGraw-Hill.

Obstetrics and Gynecology

Cunningham, F. G., Gant, N. F., Leveno, K. J., Gilstrap, L. C., Hauth, J. C., Wenstrom, K. D., eds. 2001. William's Obstetrics. 21st ed. New York: McGraw-Hill.

DeCherney, A. H., Nathan, L. 2002. Current Obstetrics and Gynecologic Diagnosis and Treatment. 9th ed. New York: McGraw-Hill.

Danforth, D. N., Gibbs, R. S., Karlan, B. Y., Haney, A. F. 2003. Danforth's Obstetrics and Gynecology. 9th ed. Baltimore, Maryland: Lippincott Williams & Wilkins.

Pediatrics

Behrman, R. E., Kliegman R. M., Jenson, H. B., eds. 2003. Nelson's Book of Pediatrics. 17th ed. Philadelphia, Pennsylvania: W. B. Saunders, Co.

Hay, W. W., Hayward, A. R., Levin, M. J., Sondheimer, J. M. 2000. Current Pediatric Diagnosis and Treatment. 15th ed. New York: McGraw-Hill.

Rudolph, C. D., Rudolph, A. M., Hostetter, M. K., Lister, G. E., Siegel, N. J., eds. 2002. Rudolph's Pediatrics. 21st ed. New York: McGraw-Hill.

Psychiatry

American Psychiatric Association. 2000. Diagnostic and Statistical Manual of Mental Disorders. (DSM-IV-TR). 4th ed. Washington, D.C.: American Psychiatric Association.

Sadock, B. J., Sadock, V. A. 2002. Kaplan and Sadock's Comprehensive Textbook of Psychiatry. 9th ed. Baltimore, Maryland: Lippincott Williams & Wilkins.

Surgery

Schwartz, S. I., Shires, G. T., Daly, J. M., eds. 1999. Principles of Surgery. 7th ed. New York: McGraw-Hill.

Way, L. W., Doherty, G. M. 2002. Current Surgical Diagnosis and Treatment. 11th ed. New York: McGraw-Hill.

Index